14.95

D1607661

# Neuro-Immune Fatigue
# ME/ CFS/FM
# And Cellular Hypoxia

David S. Bell MD, FAAP

WingSpan Press

Printed in the United States of America

Published by WingSpan Press, Livermore, CA
www.wingspanpress.com

The WingSpan name, logo and colophon are the trademarks of
WingSpan Publishing.

ISBN 978-1-59594-179-4

First edition 2007

Library of Congress Control Number 2007931521

This book is dedicated to Molly and my many patients
with Chronic Fatigue Syndrome who have taught me
the meaning of courage.


June, 2007

# Table of Contents

Introduction ............................................................ i

1: An Illness of Cellular Hypoxia .......................................... 1

2: Overview ............................................................ 7

3: Infection as the Initiating Event ....................................... 13

4: Non-Infectious Causes .................................................. 24

5: Genetic Influences ..................................................... 34

6: The Immune-Cytokine Cascade ............................................ 39

7: Nitric Oxide Metabolism ................................................ 49

8: Cluster #1 – Vasculopathy .............................................. 57

9: Cluster #2 – Central  Sensitization ..................................... 68

10: Cluster #3 – Cellular Hypoxia ......................................... 74

11: Treatment Considerations .............................................. 83

*Neuro-Immune Fatigue*
*ME/ CFS/FM*
*And Cellular Hypoxia*

# Introduction

This monograph is about chronic fatigue syndrome, myalgic encephalomyelitis or encephalopathy and fibromyalgia. And chronic Lyme disease. And chemical sensitivities. And the Tapanui flu and Lyndonville chronic mononucleosis. In 1988 I wrote a book entitled The Disease of a Thousand Names. Now it is up to two thousand names, but still the same illness. Or rather the various names refer to conditions of the same spectrum of illnesses. For the purposes of this monograph, I will call it the neuro-immune fatigue spectrum of illnesses, and it contains CFS, ME, CFIDS, FM, MCS as well as illnesses such as orthostatic intolerance, generalized migraine, chronic Lyme and many others. Or ME/CFS/FM.

The illness whose mechanism I will attempt to describe is defined as:

1) Severe, activity-limiting exhaustion, fatigue, and/or orthostatic intolerance
2) Chronic, widespread pain
3) Post-exertional malaise, or worsening of symptoms after exertion
4) Normal routine blood tests and x-rays.

ME/CFS/FM exists as an illness spectrum, with the varying colors of this spectrum being variations in the symptom complex. Each variation has stimulated its own family of descriptive names and titles, so many that the purpose of assigning a name to an illness has been lost. If this continues we will have to adopt the method used in the human genome project for naming genes: U25aP, COMT, G1743M, etc.

In this book I will not be discussing the basics of neuro-immune fatigue or ME/CFS/FM such as the clinical presentation, symptoms, prognosis and standard treatment. This monograph is not an introductory book, it is not for rookies. For those of you who are looking for an introductory book, there are several available in your local bookstore. Consider this a graduate studies level monograph.

I have chosen to write this monograph in an overly simplified style. It is designed to stimulate thinking, generate concepts, and even suggest treatment options which could lead to better patient care. If you are a primary care physician, please do not go ballistic, I mean no disrespect, as I am just a small town doctor myself. I remember when I first read Dr. Martin Pall's theory about nitric oxide in ME/CFS/FM a number of years ago (Pall-00), I said to myself that I didn't care if it was correct or incorrect, I was just too old to learn a whole new paradigm of medicine. When I went to medical school we didn't have nitric oxide. Hell, I used a slide rule in high school.

But being a clinician, I felt committed to providing medical care for my patients, many of whom have had this illness over many years. I looked for other causes of their symptoms. I tried all the standard treatments and they were disappointing. The only benefit I was to my patients was that I was able to be with them, to listen and try to fit their illness into the context of their shattered lives. And it helped a little. Nowadays it is called cognitive behavioral therapy. Whatever.

But I now see a potential for treatments and therapies that can reduce symptoms and improve daily activity. It is like one of those computer games where the hero is trundling along going through doors and windows and secret passages. Sometimes the hero stumbles on a hidden doorway that opens up into an entire universe of possibilities. Such is the situation that seems to have occurred in the science of neuro-immune fatigue, and this world revolves around cellular metabolism, nitric oxide, free radicals and oxidative damage. It results in cellular hypoxia. It is not a new science; we all studied the Krebs cycle in medical school years ago. We know a lot about it. In heart disease we are trying like mad to increase nitric oxide in order to increase blood flow to heart muscle. The tools and the science are there.

But neuro-immune fatigue is an area poorly treated by allopathic (regular) physicians. Allopathic medicine is "ritual-driven" medicine, algorithms, pre-approval certification visits and so on. Nurse practitioners and physician assistants had been trying to copy allopathic doctors, but are, fortunately, now coming into their own. I think they provide better medical care in chronic illness than their bosses. I see many ME/CFS/FM patients where the office physician has no role in managing their symptoms, as they still view this illness as a form of hysteria. But the non-physician medical providers are listening to their patients, reading, learning......

The world of medicine is changing. We are standing at a crossroads we have not seen since the 1940's when antibiotics emerged to control infectious disease. This crossroads is the point where in order to treat chronic illness we must look inside the cell, not just cover over organ related symptoms. And nowhere is this crossroads more apparent than in the leper colonies of ME/CFS/FM. Let us hope that the children of today will see neuro-immune fatigue when they become adults as infrequently as we now see persons with leprosy.

One final word. I see this monograph as a first draft. I place the date on the cover – 2007 – because in 2008 we will know so much more that this will be completely out of date. If I am guessing right the concepts may still stand, but the holes will be filled in. And maybe someday soon the medical profession will embrace neuro-immune fatigue as the harbinger of a new era of cellular medicine.

References

Pall M: Elevated, sustained peroxynitrite levels as the cause of chronic fatigue syndrome. *Med Hypotheses* 2000, 54:115-125.

# Chapter 1: An Illness of Cellular Hypoxia

For many years, persons with neuro-immune fatigue, ME/CFS/FM/FM have wandered like orphans in the world of medical providers looking for a medical specialty - any medical specialty - to take care of them. Primary care providers do not have the time and ME/CFS/FM is too complicated. Neurologists take care of multiple sclerosis patients and send ME/CFS/FM patients to psychiatrists even though the symptoms are similar. Endocrinologists do not like it because the endocrine problems originate in the brain. Gastroenterologists may look at the stomach problems but not the rest. Cardiologists measure and count palpitations and sometimes do a tilt table test but do not address the whole picture. No one has figured out what clinical ecologists do yet.

Without a medical provider to look after the ME/CFS/FM patient, the world becomes more harsh and cruel, as if the illness were not bad enough to start with. Disability issues are not met, and treatment attempts stop with the first round of antidepressants. There are hundreds of protocols available on the web, but it is too confusing for exhausted persons with cognitive difficulties to sort through. Furthermore, many of the protocols require prescriptions and the primary care physician is not going to do this for protocols and medications which make no sense. Where is the ME/CFS/FM patient to go? The problem is one of focus, and the world of medical providers needs to adjust to this change in focus in order to adapt, survive, and begin to provide basic, adequate medical care.

Traditionally, disease has been organized into categories according to the organ system that dominates the illness. Pneumonia is thought of as a lung disease. Stomach ulcers are illnesses of the digestive tract. AIDS is a "two organ disease", an infectious disease that causes a defective immune system. Multiple sclerosis is a brain disease. Psychosis is a psychiatric problem. This system of categorizing an illness by its primary organ system has never worked in neuro-immune fatigue.

In the 1950's, ME/CFS/FM was felt to be an infectious disease. Then came the notion that it was a psychiatric disease, a form of depression or hysteria that has survived the last fifty years. With the uncovering of the many neuro-endocrine abnormalities such as abnormal cortisol, growth hormone, and antidiuretic hormone, it was felt to be an endocrine disease. The bowel symptoms suggested an illness of the gastrointestinal tract. Since the 1990's, the brain has been the primary center of attention, but this has been unsatisfactory for a number of reasons. A "fatigue center" of the brain has been proposed but this was never very successful. Pain and orthostatic intolerance are neurologic but are diverse and seemingly unrelated.

It has become increasingly apparent that ME/CFS/FM is not an organ-specific illness; it is not localized in a single organ system. This method of classifying illness has never worked and remains the primary reason that ME/CFS/FM lives as an orphan. The pathology is present in every organ of the body, or more specifically, in every cell of the body. We need to change the focus of our telescope from looking at large organs to looking at single cells. And perhaps the focus needs to change even further, down to specific parts of the cell. Neuro-immune fatigue is an illness characterized by deficient cellular energy production.

Recent studies are showing that the root of the problem can be found in smooth muscle cells, brain cells, liver cells, peripheral neurons, skeletal muscle cells, heart muscle cells, and immune system cells. It is a defect so global that it cannot be adequately consigned to one type of cell, for example a nerve cell or liver cell. The difficulty in producing energy for use in the body is experienced by all the cells in all the organs. Some organs are more energy critical, and therefore stand out, the brain for example.

Concept of Hypoxia

Hypoxia is a technical term meaning the inability to transform oxygen into energy. Most frequently it refers to not getting enough oxygen to the lungs, or not getting enough oxygen into the blood stream once it reaches the lungs. A person becomes hypoxic while drowning or with lung damage as in emphysema. Hypoxia also occurs if there is a problem delivering the blood to the tissues, even though there is plenty of oxygen in the air and lungs. When blood vessels are blocked with a blood clot, the downstream tissues become "hypoxic".

However, there is a fourth type of hypoxia, and it is this fourth type that is the focus of this monograph. In this form of hypoxia, there is plenty of oxygen in the air, plenty of oxygen in the blood, and the blood gets to the tissues. This fourth type is called "cellular hypoxia" and it is due to a problem at the cellular level converting oxygen into energy.

To my knowledge, the term was first coined by Dr. Mitchell Fink referring to the problem of septic shock (Fink-97). He reviewed the series of events occurring in septic shock: first, a serious infection. Next, the infection stimulates the production of cytokines. These cytokines, while trying to fight the infection, increase the amount of nitric oxide produced within the cell. This nitric oxide then interferes with the production of energy, to the degree that a person can die of septic shock even though oxygen is given and blood is flowing to the organs. In severe septic shock the impairment of energy production by nitric oxide is similar to the effect of cyanide.

ME/CFS/FM is different from septic shock. But, is it possible that a similar mechanism, albeit slower and chronic, may be taking place? Neuro-immune fatigue may just be a minor and chronic form of septic shock. The remainder of this monograph will explore this concept and present the evidence accumulated that there is a series of events which end up disrupting the energy production cycle, and thus produce the symptoms which exist within this spectrum of illnesses.

Every illness can be looked at as a defect of cellular energy production, and there is a danger of over focusing on the cell. If a person is shot in the heart, blood drains out and oxygen cannot be delivered to the vital organs. The body's death results from the cumulative cell death from inability to convert oxygen to energy. Is this an appropriate way to classify a gunshot wound? Obviously it is not, even though it may be correct.

Abnormal metabolic pathways, faults in the cellular ability to metabolize food and oxygen to make energy, are known to occur in hundreds of illnesses. Evidence is mounting that it is of great importance in schizophrenia, autism, heart failure, renal disease and hundreds of others. Yet these illnesses are very different from one another. With ME/CFS/FM, and the lack of a dominant organ to blame the illness on, we may be witnessing the emergence of the next era of medicine: diagnosis and treatment of cellular metabolic illnesses.

## Mitochondria

Of course there have been examples of metabolic disease before. Certain illnesses have been known to be caused by disease within the mitochondria, the little power plants within cells. There are from two hundred to a thousand mitochondria in the different cells of the body. They look like round dinner tables scattered throughout a huge ballroom banquet. They do the main work of converting the oxygen we breathe in and the glucose we eat into carbon dioxide and ATP, the storage form of energy. Everything we do requires energy. Muscle contraction requires energy; making proteins in the liver requires energy; thinking requires energy. Even breaking down foodstuffs and removing toxins requires energy. It seems hard to believe that fatigue science has taken so long to get to this point. We have studied amoebae for years and understand the energy cycles very well. Is it too far a stretch to think that these systems can go wrong and cause clinical illness on a large scale in people?

## Mitochondrial myopathy

There are specific illnesses known as mitochondrial myopathies. These illnesses are, in general, very severe and often fatal. The prominent symptoms are neurologic and are usually diagnosed in early childhood. Of interest is a case report of a patient with mitochondrial myopathy who was mistakenly diagnosed with fibromyalgia (DeSouza-04). This indicates not only the need for careful diagnosis, but emphasizes the similarity between mitochondrial myopathy and illnesses with severe fatigue and widespread pain. This is becoming more true now that we can identify mitochondrial problems less severe than the fatal mitochondrial myopathies.

In a recent paper concerning gene expression in patients who have had a recent Epstein-Barr virus infection, a link to mitochondrial dysfunction was suggested. Suzanne Vernon and her co-workers

4

noted that the gene expression profile of EBV patients with persistent fatigue was different from those patients with EBV who recovered uneventfully. They noted that "several of the differentially expressed genes affect mitochondrial functions including fatty acid metabolism and the cell cycle."(Vernon-06)

We are just beginning to explore the relationship between energy production in the mitochondria and clinical illness. We still do not know if it is even appropriate to consider ME/CFS/FM primarily as a metabolic illness. But it also opens extraordinary doors with the potential for treatment. If neuro-immune fatigue is an illness caused by a defect in energy production, or several defects in energy production, correction of those defects would cause an improvement not seen to date. It is just possible that the future understanding of ME/CFS/FM treatment will make us think that treating it with antidepressants is not far removed from treating the cholera patient with blood-letting.

In this monograph, I would like to explore the concept of neuro-immune fatigue as a metabolic illness resulting from a series of events beginning with an infection, toxic exposure, or neurologic injury. These initiating events in a genetically sensitive person lead to immune system abnormalities and cause an excess production of nitric oxide or inability to eliminate it properly. Nitric oxide and/or its toxic by-products then produce the three distinct clinical abnormalities that define neuro-immune fatigue: a) blood flow and vascular abnormalities contributing to orthostatic intolerance (vasculopathy), b) widespread pain, as well as sensitivities to foods, temperature, light, noise and odors (central sensitization), and c) fatigue and exhaustion (impaired energy production). It is this third symptom cluster that takes place in the mitochondria of individual cells.

I do not wish to suggest that this is a new concept. Drs. McCully, Natelson, and co-workers published a paper in 1996 demonstrating reduced muscle oxidative metabolism, and many other papers have been published since then. It is really back to the concept of focus. People say that we do not know the cause of ME/CFS/FM. I would maintain that we actually do, but we have neglected to focus on the evidence that turns up abnormal in almost every study – the ability of the individual brain, muscle and other cells to produce adequate energy.

## References

DeSouza R, Cardenas R, TU L, De la Fuente F, Mayorquin F, Trochtenberg D: Mitochondrial encephalo-myopathy with lactic acidosis and strokelike episodes (MELAS): a mitochondrial disorder presents as fibromyalgia. *South Med J* 2004, 97:528-31.(5):528-531.

Fink M: Cytopathic hypoxia in sepsis. *Acta Anaesthesiol Scand* 1997, 41(Suppl 100):87-95.

McCully K, Natelson B, Iotti S, Sisto S, Leigh J: Reduced oxidative muscle metabolism in the chronic fatigue syndrome. *Muscle Nerve* 1996, 19:621-625.

Vernon S, Whistler T, Cameron B, Hickie I, Reeves W, Lloyd A: Preliminary evidence of mitochondrial dysfunction associated with post-infectious fatigue after acute infection with Epstein-Barr virus. *BMC Infectious Diseases* 2006, 6: http://www.biomedcentral.com/1471-2334/1476/1416.

# Chapter 2: Overview

Sometimes a concept is hard to grasp because it is just too simple. This may be the case with neuro-immune fatigue. For example, take fatigue that is caused by fasting. A healthy person begins a three day fast, or is thrown into a dungeon without food. After a while, that person begins to get hungry, and then weak. In a couple of days the weakness and exhaustion is so severe it is hard to move around. Yet the person does not look particularly ill.

In this case, the origin of the fatigue is not hard to figure out; it is lack of food. When this person is given food, he or she returns to normal strength, thus confirming our suspicion. The fatigue was caused by the lack of food (glucose) and because of its lack, it could not be turned into energy (ATP). In an oversimplified diagram, it would look like this:

$$\text{Glucose} \quad + \quad \text{Oxygen} \quad \longrightarrow \quad \text{Carbon Dioxide} \quad + \quad \text{ATP}$$

The oxygen in the air we breathe is used metabolically with glucose to produce energy as stored in ATP. The carbon dioxide we breathe out is a by-product. All this takes place in the mitochondria. There. All of high school biology in one paragraph. The main reason I like to oversimplify things is that I failed high school biology.

As discussed in the last chapter, this process is called oxidative metabolism. Metabolism is defined as the chemical changes within cells and for our purposes we will be talking mostly about those changes requiring oxygen. Our premise is that there is something wrong with this chemical process, and as a result there is a reduction in the amount of energy produced and stored in the body. It is not the same as fasting, or going without food. In that scenario, the person wastes away and gets thin like a movie star. In ME/CFS/FM the glucose is taken in but not burned so it gets stored as fat. Because there is not enough ATP produced, there is not enough energy produced to go and jog it off.

The next part of the process is to examine why this oxidative metabolism is not working properly. And here we need to talk about the chain of events that takes place between the ingestion of food and the production of energy. This chain of events is enormously complex with many steps. Any one of those steps that is missing or damaged can cause a disruption of the process of energy production. A big disruption or major break in the chain is fatal because without energy the body cannot survive. But with more subtle chemical injuries, like what is likely going on in neuro-immune fatigue, the body manages to get enough energy to survive, and maybe even walk around for a few hours a day, but not enough to feel well.

This chain of events in the process of oxidative metabolism has hundreds of different chemical reactions taking place. Scholars and scientists have not accepted the existence of ME/CFS/FM because they say it is not one illness, it is "heterogeneous", and they are correct. The disruption in the normal matabolic chain is likely to occur in different places for different people, and here is where it gets almost hopelessly complicated. Science is just beginning to tackle this area with genomic and metabolic studies. But the diagnosis of neuro-immune fatigue as a spectrum is useful because it encompasses the whole chain.

We can break it down further. We know it is a process not confined to one cell type such as muscle or nerve. It is different from cyanide poisoning, cardiomyopathy, and septic shock, and we know the clinical events that define ME/CFS/FM. Combining the knowledge of clinical events, individual scientific studies within ME/CFS/FM, and an understanding of normal physiology, we could hypothesize a chain of events that looks like this:

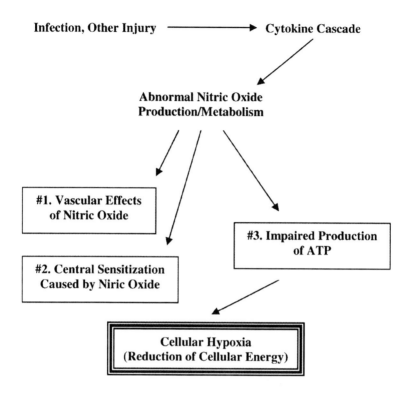

This diagram will serve as a template for the chapters to follow. The initial insults of the illness cause an abnormal immunologic cascade which affects the basic cellular metabolism of nitric oxide. The abnormalities here lead to the three symptom clusters that characterize the illness – vascular, central sensitization and impaired energy production. And central to all three symptom clusters lies nitric oxide.

Nitric oxide

Nitric oxide is a tiny molecule that is at the core of huge numbers of processes that take place within the cell. It is an important part of the chain of events resulting in energy production, or rather, it plays an important part in the disruption of the energy production process. As first described by Drs. Martin Pall, Paul Cheney, Kenny DeMeirleir, and others several years ago, disruptions in the nitric oxide pathways poison the energy production pathways and produce the symptoms of neuro-immune fatigue.

But nitric oxide is critical to the survival of every cell in our body; it cannot be thought of as bad or evil. It is not our enemy. Like anything else, if over-produced it can cause problems. It has the normal functions of helping to regulate blood flow and blood vessel diameter, functioning normally as a vasodilator. This means that it affects blood flow to the brain and plays a role in orthostatic problems. It is necessary for memory formation and normal apoptosis, or programmed cell death. It affects natural killer cell function and immunity. It is a neurotransmitter in certain situations. It modulates or modifies neuroendocrine functions, and it is important in cell metabolism. An over production of nitric oxide or problems in its metabolite degradation leads to an excess of the toxic metabolites that poison mitochondria. Overall, this excess leads to three symptom clusters.

Vasculopathy (our #1 in the scheme above) is a general term meaning abnormal functioning of the vascular system. We know this occurs in ME/CFS/FM with studies showing changes in blood pressure, tissue blood flow, brain blood flow, and orthostatic intolerance. The vasculopathy can lead to symptoms mediated directly by abnormal blood flow, such as headache, cognitive disturbance, and orthostatic intolerance. The body may try to compensate for abnormal blood flow by over-secreting adrenalin, causing the "frazzled" or "wired and tired" sensation, as well as causing measurable changes in the neuro-endocrine system.

Central sensitization is a general term referring to a hyper-sensitivity of the sensory apparatus of the central nervous system. The central sensitization of neuro-immune fatigue results in increased sensory perception and leads to great distress. For the ME/CFS/FM patient, it is experienced as pain, tender points, headache, and sensitivity to light, noise, odors, and chemicals. I is likely to contribute to the lymph node pain and sore throat.

But the biggest problem, hiding in plain sight, are the symptoms of our cluster #3, a reduction of energy production. It is called cellular hypoxia, a defect in oxidative phosphorylation. It is a defect that prevents oxygen from being effectively converted to energy. It is perceived by the patient as fatigue, weakness, abnormal gastrointestinal motility, cognitive problems, sleep problems, and post-exertional malaise. It is this area that makes the life of persons with ME/CFS/FM very miserable indeed.

Left out of this scheme are other effects of nitric oxide excess such as changes in platelet aggregation, apoptosis, and the immune system. There are so many effects of excess nitric oxide that it is nearly impossible to put them into discrete categories. With each effect studied, we have a different perspective of the illness. Neuro-immune fatigue has also been called the low natural killer cell syndrome, generalized migraine, multiple chemical sensitivities, and so on.

This is the premise to be explored in the following chapters. Time will tell if it is correct, or even close. But if the nitric oxide pathway is the culprit in ME/CFS/FM, then finding the specific defect in this pathway for a particular individual will lead to a correction of that defect. This approach was adopted in hematology in the area of bleeding disorders. In the 18th century the only treatment for bleeding was to apply a bandage. Science has led us to an understanding of the many specific abnormalities in the blood clotting pathway, and now we can give a platelet transfusion to persons with missing platelets, or Factor IX to someone with hemophilia. Unfortunately for most persons with ME/CFS/FM, at the present time the bandage is the only therapy available.

## Summary

#1. Illness Onset. Roughly 75% of ME/CFS/FM begins with an infection. But other events may initiate the illness such as toxic exposure, physical and mental stress, head injury or other types of neurologic injury. In short neuro-immune fatigue can be initiated by anything that affects the nitric oxide pathway.

#2. The Cytokine Cascade. After an initiating infection, a cytokine cascade occurs. Cytokines are chemicals such as interferon, interleukins and many others which, while helping you fight the infection, make you feel sick while they are doing their job. In healthy persons the cytokine cascade shuts down after the infection is conquered, and the person returns to good health. In ME/CFS/FM this does not occur and the chain of events continues to unravel.

#3. <u>Gene Transcription.</u> The cytokine cascade initiates protein messengers and gene transcription factors that communicate with genetic material, RNA and DNA. Very complicated, lets ignore it for now.

#4. <u>Nitric Oxide Synthetase enzyme.</u> This causes the enzyme iNOS to become active. This enzyme, called inducible Nitric Oxide Synthetase, makes nitric oxide out of L-arginine. There are other forms of this enzyme, but the end result is that an excess of nitric oxide is produced.

#5. <u>Excess Nitric Oxide.</u> An excess of nitric oxide causes two sets of problems. First there is an exaggerated response due to too much nitric oxide doing what it normally does, and this leads to the blood vessel problems and pain. The second problem is that the by-products of nitric oxide production, called reactive oxygen species (ROS), superoxide, and peroxynitrite, are increased. These are the main suspects in the mitochondrial poisoning process. Variations in symptom expression from person to person within the illness spectrum can be due to the large number of steps involved and an individual's genetic make-up.

#6. <u>Disruption of Energy Production.</u> Either nitric oxide itself or its by-products interfere with oxidative phosphorylation in the mitochondria and cause cellular hypoxia. This disruption leads to a decreased production of ATP. Some of this disruption is likely to be permanent and cannot be corrected unless new healthy mitochondria are manufactured. Some disruption is reversible and will be reversed by rest.

# Chapter 3: Infection as the Initiating Event

While the question of what causes ME/CFS/FM is logically the first question on people's mind, it is almost an inappropriate question. It has occupied many years of research on the illness, and has caused enormous confusion, yet now fades to the background because it is becoming apparent that it is almost irrelevant. The difficulty in finding "a cause" has been one of the prime reasons that people have doubted the reality of this illness. What has become apparent is that there are many "causes"; what is important now is not so much the initiating event or infection, but the mechanism of what perpetuates the illness. In other words, it is not the actual onset that matters, but why the symptoms do not resolve after the onset.

The confusion relates to the fact that the initiating factors for ME/CFS/FM are commonplace. Every day patients come into my office with something that can begin the nightmare of ME/CFS/FM. Fortunately, the vast majority of persons resolve their problem and never come to know of this nightmare that could have been.

I would estimate that there may be more than ten causes of the process we are calling ME/CFS/FM. But for the sake of simplicity, let us restrict ourselves to just a few. The first in this list would be infection. It is the classic presentation of a previously healthy person who develops a commonplace mononucleosis, sinus infection, or bronchitis and never gets better. That seventy five percent of all persons with ME/CFS/FM begin this way is a reasonable guess. The remaining will initiate their illness with head injury, other types of neurologic injury, toxic exposure, or some type of stress. For some, the illness comes on gradually without a clear initiating event.

Assessing the cause is much more difficult than it would seem. It is human nature to seek explanations, and sometimes we will be happy with an explanation even if it is wrong. It has been my experience that when I ask a patient how the illness began, they will say, "with a fever, on January 18th." On further questioning, however, they had been tired and run down for weeks before, and had recently developed migraine headaches and irritable bowel. Perhaps the episode of fever merely pointed out a process well underway already.

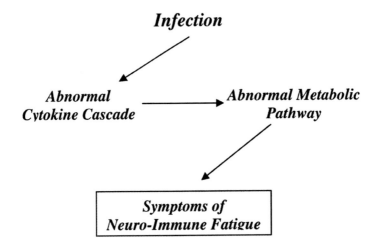

Infection is the first of the causes we will examine here. The infection may be due to a virus (hence the older term "post-viral fatigue"), or it may be due to a parasite, bacteria, rickettsia, or other type of infectious organism. There have been many organisms so far that have been implicated in initiating the chain of evens that results in neuro-immune fatigue. It appears that the critical factor is not the initiating infection but rather the steps which occur immediately after the infection, the cascade of immune chemicals called cytokines.

This cascade of cytokines, to be described in a later chapter, is different in those persons who recover uneventfully from the infection, as opposed to those persons who go on to develop ME/CFS/FM. It is not unusual to hear someone say, "Four people in the family got ill with a virus, but the other three got well within a week. Mine has stayed for six years." The initiating virus was not the real problem, it was how and why the person with neuro-immune fatigue responded to it.

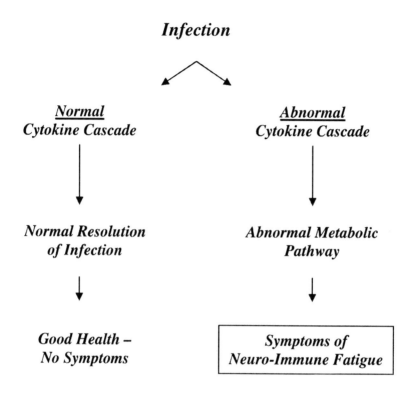

It can be difficult to identify the initiating infection. By the time you diagnose neuro-immune fatigue at six months of illness, it is nearly impossible by the standard tests to find the organism. Too much time has elapsed. For a standard infection, for example, it is necessary to measure the antibodies at the beginning, before the body has made an immune response, and again at six weeks when the immune response is cranking out antibodies. This is never done in ME/CFS/FM because during the initiating infection it is assumed that it will be just another trivial virus that is going to go away by itself. As one of my patients said in disgust, "just another damn virus." Soon technologies will be available to look for viral load, to measure the actual amount of a specific virus in the body, and not just the body's immune response to it. If the initiating infection goes away and the process or chain of events causing ME/CFS/FM continues, it will not matter what the initiating infection was. However, as we will discuss later, it is quite possible that the initiating infection "hangs around" and continues to perpetuate the chain of events.

This second issue has caused great confusion. Does the infection that starts ME/CFS/FM go away after initiating a process which causes the illness, (a "hit and run" onset) or is the illness due to a persisting infection? This is a critical question because if it is a "hit and run" illness, the damage caused by the infection cannot be treated with antibiotics or antivirals because it is too late. If ME/CFS/FM is a persistent or ongoing infection, then the antibiotic or antiviral, (if you choose the right one) will do the trick and cure the illness.

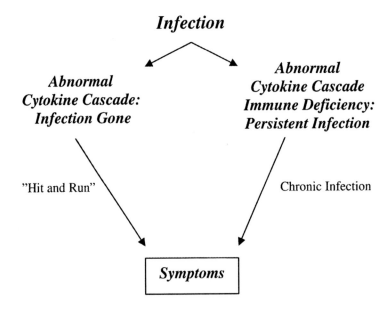

An example of both mechanisms is illustrated by the strep germ. An initial infection causes a strep throat, which may go away by itself, even without antibiotics. Sometimes there is persistent infection, an abscess in the tonsils, and this can be treated and cured by penicillin. Other times, the strep germ resolves normally but has started the process of rheumatic fever, and at a certain point giving the penicillin is not going to cure the problem because it is not simply a persistent infection. In rheumatic fever, the strep germ began a process that takes on a life of its own.

Let us look at some of the infectious agents that have been implicated in neuro-immune fatigue, with specific reference to the question of whether evidence points to either "hit and run" phenomenon or persistent infection.

Epstein-Barr virus

Long ago, what we now call ME/CFS/FM was called chronic mononucleosis. Oddly enough, fifty years later it turns out that this name was more accurate than anything we now have. We became confused when we could not identify the virus of mononucleosis (Epstein-Barr virus or EBV) causing an ongoing infection. But clinicians knew that some persons who got mono just did not recover properly. A study in Dubbo, Australia, has helped to clarify this.

In this study, researchers identified patients who came down with mononucleosis and two other infections, and followed them to see what happened. The majority had an unpleasant time for a few weeks and then started to improve with complete recovery within a month or so. However, of the 101 persons with Epstein-Barr virus mononucleosis, six percent developed neuro-immune fatigue one year later. The most important predictor of developing the illness was the severity of the initiating infection, and neither emotions nor history of psychiatric problems was a factor (Hickie-06). For these persons, it can be said that mononucleosis, or rather the Epstein-Barr virus, was the cause of their neuro-immune fatigue.

The next part of this study is more important. The investigators looked at the differences that existed between those people who had a regular course of mononucleosis, and those who went on to develop ME/CFS/FM. While all the answers are far from in, there appears to be a specific series of events that takes place that causes the persistence of illness in some persons. Understanding this process is critical to interrupting it, and we will be discussing this process in the other chapters.

In past years the attempts to treat ME/CFS/FM have revolved around attempts to kill the virus or organism which has caused the illness. For example, if Epstein-Barr virus were to cause or start ME/CFS/FM, then why not treat the person with antiviral drugs to eradicate the virus? There are several good anti-viral drugs that are effective against Epstein-Barr virus, but in the past they have not worked. This may be because while EBV set off the illness, the Epstein-Barr virus has resolved by the time we attempt to treat it. It is like a hiker on the top of a mountain who kicks a rock off the edge and then walks away. The rock tumbles down the hillside, picking up speed and other rocks and starts a landslide. The hiker walks back to his car and hears about the landslide on the evening news.

However, in the 2007 IACFS meetings a paper presented by a group at Stanford was obtaining good results with a potent anti-viral drug that targeted EBV. Potentially very good news, but at the time of this writing it is premature to make this conclusion.

<u>Poliomyelitis</u>

EBV is one infectious agent that has been associated with neuro-immune fatigue, but there are many others. Historically the enterovirus family of viruses has been connected to the development of the illness and has been the center of interest in the UK ever since the Royal Free Hospital outbreak in 1950. Poliovirus belongs to this family and is well known to cause post-infectious fatigue, known as the post-polio syndrome.

There are two separate difficulties that come from infection with the poliovirus. First is damage to the spinal cord which results in acute paralysis; it is this which the infection is noted for and which caused the widespread panic in the 1950's. Second is the "post-polio syndrome" characterized by exhaustion, progressive muscle weakness, pain, and other symptoms. It is likely that the post polio syndrome is due to damage to the midbrain that does not become fully apparent for some time. However, it appears that the poliovirus itself is cleared by the immune system whether or not damage is done. The later problems are unlikely to be due to a persistent infection.

Other enteroviruses, and there are many, have been implicated in ME/CFS/FM for over twenty years. During the period that this was being studied most intensely, an understanding of the immune response, or cascade initiated by the infection, was in its infancy. Most of the research placed an emphasis on looking for remnants of the virus in muscle tissue. Interestingly, these remnants can be found in a large percentage of neuro-immune fatigue patients. This may imply increased presence, or even chronic enteroviral infection.

Parvovirus

Parvovirus is an exceptionally interesting candidate to cause both ME/CFS/FM, and the evidence is in conflict as to whether this "cause" is from the initiation of a cytokine cascade or from persistent infection. This is an important candidate to study in that parvovirus B19 infection may cause no symptoms at all, a minor infection, or prolonged complications, including persistent fatigue, muscle pain, anemia, arthritis, heart muscle infection, and other problems. How this virus can do this is critical to know.

Jonathon Kerr and co-workers have noted that 10% to 15% of parvovirus B19 patients developed chronic fatigue syndrome, and up to 60% developed fibromyalgia. On standard testing, these patients appeared as if they had cleared the initiating infection effectively despite having persistent symptoms. Importantly, one patient with ME/CFS/FM that developed from parvovirus B19 infection had no antibodies at all against it one year after developing neuro-immune fatigue. This means that it is unreliable to look for parvovirus once the acute infection has resolved. However, persistent fatigue was associated with the presence of gamma interferon and tumor necrosis factor alpha. This would imply that symptom persistence would be related to the immune activation and the presence of cytokines, a cytokine cascade.

However they also did a couple of other things. They looked at the pro-inflammatory cytokines, and attempted to see if there was an abnormality in the genetic makeup of an individual who had persistence of symptoms after infection. They found that one gene in particular (Ku80 gene) was abnormal. This gene happens to be a B19 co-receptor. Therefore, this would give a potential mechanism for virus persistence and ongoing infection. In addition, they published three cases of persistent chronic fatigue treated with intravenous gamma globulin which resolved persistent B19 in the blood, the cytokine dysregulation, as well as the symptoms of ME/CFS/FM.

There are several take home messages from their studies. First, this virus may "cause" both chronic fatigue syndrome and fibromyalgia, strengthening the link between these conditions. Secondly, if you can find parvovirus as an initiating infection and if you find persistence of this virus in the blood stream, there may be an effective treatment, but this requires aggressive clinical management starting from the first week of severe fatigue. Thirdly, if no investigations had been carried out during the first two years of illness, it may be impossible to detect parvovirus B19 even if it had initiated the illness.

## Q fever

Q fever happens to be one of my personal favorites in the study of infections which initiate neuro-immune fatigue for strictly personal reasons. I had the good fortune to visit Professor Barry Marmion in 1987 in Australia and see a few of his "Post Q fever" patients who looked exactly like my patients in Lyndonville. My patients had been exposed to unpasturized milk but did not have Q fever. Dr. Marmion's patients had classical Q fever and had been treated properly right from the beginning.

Q fever is an infection caused by Coxiella brunetti which is not a virus but a rickettsia, and is an occupational hazard for abattoir workers in Australia. The infection is carried in sheep and after processing lamb for market, some persons get Q fever. It has been well recognized and well treated in Australia for years.

At first, when cases did not seem to resolve normally despite appropriate antibiotic treatment, the government felt the workers were "faking it" in order to collect unemployment. Sound familiar? However, two managers developed the "post Q fever debility syndrome" and they were not eligible for unemployment benefits. The government then became interested and began a series of studies with Dr. Marmion. It is now clear that more than 5% of persons with Q fever, even those who were treated well at the onset of their infection, go on to develop ME/CFS/FM.

## Lyme disease

Lyme disease has its controversial side, and it is not surprising that it fits in this discussion of ME/CFS/FM. As an acute illness, Lyme is known for its rash, neurologic and rheumatologic symptoms, and a percentage of persons who get Lyme disease do not recover. It is caused by a spirochete, Borrelia burgdorferi, and, unlike viruses, it is an organism that can be cured with antibiotics. The crucial question that plagues the subject of chronic Lyme disease is whether the illness is due to persistence of the organism, or is it a "hit and run" illness? If it is entirely due to persisting infection, it should be treatable with high dose antibiotics.

At present there are anecdotal reports that long term antibiotics have been successful in the treatment of ME/CFS/FM, but it should be remembered that a substantial number of persons with the illness get better by themselves in the first few years of the illness. That means that if someone is quite ill at two years of illness and begins either antibiotics or vitamins or any other treatment, they have nearly an 80% chance of getting better over the next two years regardless of the treatment. However if someone is still ill at five years, it is unlikely that they will improve spontaneously.

Personally, I have not had success with long term antibiotics in my patients.

Other

There are many other infections implicated in starting ME/CFS/FM, and each of them has its own supporters. In the past, studies have shown that each of them is not "the cause", meaning that there is not a large enough block of one initiating infection to make a statistical dent if looked at a whole population.

In Lyndonville, for instance, there was an outbreak in 1985, and I was certain that one specific virus or bacteria set it off. I feel this way because the appearance of the first few weeks was nearly the same from person to person. This is different from the patients I see now from different areas in the country who have had their ME/CFS/FM initiated in a variety of different ways.

Other legitimate contenders for the honorary title of neuro-immune fatigue cause include Brucella, Ross River virus, Hepatitis C, mycoplasma, Inoue-Melnick virus, and Borna virus. I have one patient whose illness began after documented Histoplasmosis and another after psittacosis. There is likely a huge range of infectious agents that have the potential to cause the illness. We need to establish what these particular infections have in common which can set off ME/CFS/FM in susceptible persons.

Conclusions

Infection is likely to be the most common way that neuro-immune fatigue begins. It is likely that people who get the illness have an infection just like other members of their family, but their immune system does not resolve this infection. It continues to produce chemicals called cytokines, which cause the person to feel ill even though the initiating infection may go away. Alternatively, there may be persistence of the infection in the patient, but at a level that is difficult to detect.

It is possible that both mechanisms occur at the same time. The original infection initiates a process that both causes symptoms and impairs immunity so that the initiating organism may linger.

The implications of this are straightforward. First it is necessary to know which infection began the illness, and this means early recognition of neuro-immune fatigue. Testing for specific initiating infections should occur if someone has a particularly severe first three weeks of illness, or is still ill at one month after an infection. It is not appropriate to waste this time by saying that a person who has not recovered at three weeks may have had a childhood emotional trauma that has turned him or her into a whiner.

Secondly, treatment should be aggressive, and directed toward the initiating infection early in the course of the illness, perhaps beginning as early as three weeks into the illness. And thirdly, medications which can disrupt the abnormal cascade of cytokines should be sought, but this must be done carefully because of potential immunologic complications.

As we will discuss in the next chapter, infection is not the only cause of neuro-immune fatigue. But I suspect that there is a common mechanism that leads to the persistence of the symptoms through this whole spectrum of conditions.

## References

Cairns V, Godwin J. Post-Lyme borreliosis syndrome: a meta-analysis of reported symptoms. Int J Epidemiol. 2005;34:1340-1345.

Chia JK. The role of enterovirus in chronic fatigue syndrome. J Clin Pathol. 2005;58:1126-1132.

Hickie I, Davenport T, Wakefield D, Vollmer-Conna U, Cameron B, Vernon S, Reeves W, Lloyd A: Post-infective and chronic fatigue syndromes precipitated by viral and non-viral pathogens: prospective cohort study. *BMJ* 2006, doi:10.1136/bmj.38933.585764.AE.

Kerr J, Cunniffe V, Kelleher P, Bernstein R, Bruce I. Successful intravenous immunoglobulin therapy in 3 cases of parvovirus B19-associated chronic fatigue syndrome. Clin Inf Dis 2003;36:e100-e106

Kerr JR, Cunniffe VS, Kelleher P, Coats AJ, Mattey DL. Circulating cytokines and chemokines in acute symptomatic parvovirus B19 infection: negative association between levels of pro-inflammatory cytokines and development of B-19 associated arthritis. J Med Virol 2004; 74 (1):147-155.

Kerr JR. Pathogenesis of parvovirus B19 infection: host gene variability, and possible means and effects of virus persistence. J Vet Med B Infect Dis Vet Public Health. 2005; 52(7-8):335-339.

Kerr JR, Barah F, Mattey DL, Laing I, Hopkins SJ, Hutchinson IV, Tyrrell DAJ. Circulating tumor necrosis factor-a and interferon-g are detectable during acute and convalescent parvovirus B19 infection and are associated with prolonged and chronic fatigue.

White P, Thomas J, Sullivan R, Buchwald D. The nosology of sub-acute and chronic fatigue syndromes that follow infectious mononucleosis. Psychol. Med. 2004;34:499-507.

# Chapter 4: Non-Infectious Causes

Infections are not the only cause of neuro-immune fatigue, and this has been another area of confusion. Of course we are referring to the whole spectrum of neuro-immune fatigue as some of the individual conditions are named for the method of onset – post-concussive syndrome, for example. By viewing infectious onset alongside non-infectious causes a broader picture is possible; it is better than splitting hairs and having two thousand separate diagnoses. Subgrouping and micro classifying can be left to the researchers.

In the last chapter we discussed the role of infections or other antigenic stimuli such as vaccinations as the cause of up to 75% of ME/CFS/FM. The remaining 25% of cases are initiated not by infections, but by some other event that sets in motion the chain of events leading to the symptom pattern. As time goes on there will be defined subgroups to neuro-immune fatigue, and it may be that at some point we will be able to do specific testing that will identify these subgroups. It is likely that the different subgroups will require different treatments as well.

At this point, however, it looks as if a similar pattern of events occurs after the initiating event, whether infectious or not. If so, it may turn out that the initiating event, even though it defines subgroups, will be irrelevant. An example of this latter concept is the common cold, where there are hundreds of different viral causes, but the illness looks the same regardless of which specific virus happens to be the culprit.

Again, we are arguing here that the mechanism generating symptoms is roughly the same whether ME/CFS/FM is set off by an infectious agent or some other event. But whatever sets the steps in motion, the paths merge at a point prior to the production of cellular energy. From that point on, the steps are relatively uniform, regardless of cause. This is illustrated in the following figure, and the steps that occur after the paths merge, the abnormal metabolic pathways, will be discussed for the bold reader in the chapters that follow.

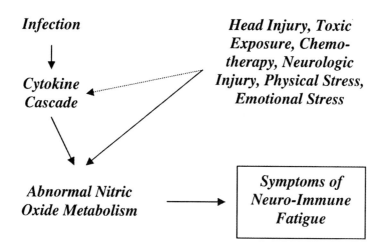

I have heard physicians say that ME/CFS/FM does not exist as a specific illness because practically everything can cause it. That is like saying that cancer does not exist. When a medical provider says this, patients "hear" that the providers do not believe in the existence of fatigue, when it really means that it is so common that the providers do not concentrate on it. The two mistakes that health care providers make is that when they do not find a specific disease/cause for the symptoms (for example a specific allergy), they ignore the symptoms, illness, and the patient. Secondly, they do not understand the impact of these symptoms, particularly the activity limitation and post-exertional malaise, on the life of a person with ME/CFS/FM.

We will start our review of the non-infectious causes with a discussion of MS and other classical neurologic illnesses.

Multiple Sclerosis

One disease that poses a constant challenge for the clinician facing a patient with severe fatigue and neurologic symptoms is multiple sclerosis (MS). The similarities between MS and neuro-immune fatigue are remarkable. Both have fatigue, muscle pain, numbness and tingling, cognitive difficulties, and weakness. Both illnesses can be disabling. The differences include the quality and quantity of exhaustion, and the lack of "fixed" or unchanging neurologic damage in ME/CFS/FM. MS patients have fatigue, but it is a "burned out" fatigue. Orthostatic intolerance is more prominent in ME/CFS/FM. Laboratory tests, lumbar puncture, and MRI scans help to distinguish the two illnesses.

It has always been particularly frustrating for patients with ME/CFS/FM to go to the neurologist, present the symptoms and have an exam and be told that they do not have MS. The patient "hears" from the neurologist that there is "nothing wrong" because they do not have MS, when in fact the neurologist is only saying that they do not have MS. But being told to go away and see someone else, maybe a psychiatrist, is devastating for the patients with ME/CFS/FM. They would rather be told that they have a possibly fatal neurologic disease, believe it or not. It is an illustration of the importance of illness validation by a medical provider.

MS has other similarities to ME/CFS/FM. It also is initiated by an infection of some kind, and many agents have been implicated. The cytokine cascade that occurs after the infectious insult is similar as well, predominantly the class called "pro-inflammatory cytokines". Where the illnesses differ is that an injury to the blood-brain barrier in MS allows the immune system to react with nervous tissue called myelin. This is the "plaque" of MS; it is a scar that results in permanent neurologic deficits.

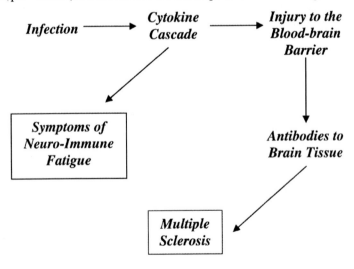

In this model, ME/CFS/FM is actually a "pre MS"; it is multiple sclerosis without the scarring and permanent damage. This is potentially good news because it would imply reversibility. While ME/CFS/FM and MS usually follow their own individual courses, some patients have "crossed over" from ME/CFS/FM to MS. Upstate New York has been called the MS capitol of the world because of the high incidence of MS, and nearly everyone else here has ME/CFS/FM. It cannot be a coincidence.

More importantly, it would be nice to know how ME/CFS/FM patients respond to the newer MS treatments, but this has never been attempted in a systematic manner. We know that there are minor responses to steroids such as prednisone in ME/CFS/FM and this has long been used in the treatment of MS. In neuro-immune fatigue however, the drawback of steroids may outweigh the benefits and they are rarely used. The new treatments are another story. Because they are expensive, risky, and ME/CFS/FM has been ignored, the cytokine altering agents have not been tried. Furthermore, because ME/CFS/FM is considered an illness of fruitcakes by medical professionals, drug companies have stayed far away from putting the serious money into treatment trials. For a review of MS, see Frohman-2006.

## Other Diseases of the Central Nervous System

One of the first lessons I learned in this topic came when a fifty year old patient, previously healthy, suffered a stroke. The patient was hospitalized and had clear neurologic deficits which located the exact position of the stroke in the brain. However, the overwhelming fatigue experienced by the patient was almost more debilitating than the stroke itself. With time the brain tissue healed somewhat but the fatigue never resolved.

I also remember that the neurologist never mentioned the fatigue in the notes as it was taken for granted – of course she had fatigue, she had a stroke. It was as irrelevant as noting that she had two ears. It is one reason that persons with ME/CFS/FM feel disrespected. Physicians, particularly neurologists, do not seem to register with the symptom of fatigue, it is just too common. It is present in just about every neurologic disease there is. For a review of the subject, please see Drs. Chaudhuri and Behan-2004.

## Head injury and Post-Concussive Syndrome

Concussion is defined as a head injury usually resulting in temporary loss of consciousness. A more accurate definition revolves around amnesia, or loss of memory, for the event. An example is the football player who runs the wrong way with the ball, but cannot remember it the next day. Most persons with concussion recover without difficulty, but some persons develop "post-concussive syndrome" characterized by fatigue, headache, diffuse pain, confusion, and difficulty concentrating. It is expected to last for a day or two, but for some persons it lasts for months and years.

A more dramatic part of this spectrum is the head injury which involves bleeding into the brain. Obviously the greater the amount of tissue damage the greater likelihood of persistent neurological damage and fatigue. But the damage is not just the bruised or killed neurons from the injury. The damage is more related to the chemical changes initiated by the injury, and it is this aspect that is the current object of immediate treatment by neurologists after a head injury or stroke. We will be delving into this subject in later chapters, as it represents the spot where the infectious and non-infectious pathways merge. The neurologic treatments designed to inhibit the chemical damage initiated by the head injury must be started immediately in order to reduce the long term damage. This, of course, is of concern because waiting the defined six months in ME/CFS/FM may be not only inappropriate but too late.

## Post-Polio Syndrome

Polio is a neurologic infection, and, as discussed in the last chapter, causes two types of damage. One is injury and cell death of tissue in the brain and in the spinal cord, resulting in paralysis. The second type of injury is the neuro-immune fatigue which can occur without any measurable damage to the nervous tissue at the time of infection (Bruno-1999). The severe fatigue that results from poliovirus infection may take years to express itself. By definition, any documented polio prior to the development of ME/CFS/FM is usually called the post-polio syndrome.

In polio we have a unique model: ME/CFS/FM can be either due to the infection of polio, (an infectious cause); it may be due to the neurologic damage caused by the infection (a non-infectious cause) or a combination of both. In fact, this is an issue that needs to be resolved in research as we often see patients with ME/CFS/FM who have had an episode of meningitis or encephalitis in the past. It is also likely that ME/CFS/FM would follow West Nile virus infection.

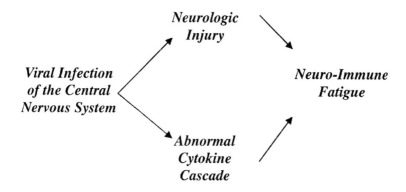

## Migraine and the Concept of Generalized Migraine

Migraine is another enormously complex subject. The common perception of migraine is that it is a nasty headache and that's it. But it is a disease characterized by recurrent bouts of headache, severe fatigue, and manifestations of central stimulus sensitization – sensitivity to sensory stimuli such as light, noise, and odors. Some persons during a migraine headache have allodynia – severe pain even to light touch all over the body. The first time I heard patients say that his or her hair hurt, I thought of migraine. Either that or the individual had vaulted over the barriers of reason and had become a fruitcake.

But sensory sensitization is a central characteristic of migraine just as it is in neuro-immune fatigue. In fact migraine is so confusing that in the back rooms of migraine conferences, battles rage not unlike those in ME/CFS/FM conferences. One expert claims that there are more than thirty subtypes of migraine. Abdominal migraine is said to be abdominal pain without the headache. The only practical difference between migraine and ME/CFS/FM is that the former is episodic; in between headaches, the migraineur feels well. The patient with ME/CFS/FM never returns to completely well although there are relapses and remissions. Some neurologists call severe daily headache with the other ME/CFS/FM symptoms "generalized migraine" or "transformed migraine." Add two more names to the list of names for neuro-immune fatigue.

In a 1995 study, we selected fifteen patients who had light-headedness and dizziness as a prominent symptom of their ME/CFS/FM. The patients were studied with sophisticated testing of the vestibular system of the brain. Their study results were suggestive of "vestibular migraine", a reduction of blood flow through the vestibular part of the brain (Ash-Bernal-1995). We will explore issues related to brain blood flow in a later chapter on the vasculopathy.

Heavy Metal Poisoning and Other Types of Brain injury

Ciguatera poisoning was shown to cause ME/CFS/FM (Pearn-2001). Once again, hopes soared that we were finally getting somewhere! I eagerly dug out the paper to find that ciguatera was a specific poison found in the puffer or blowfish in the Sea of Japan, and that if people ate it raw (as in sushi) they could get ME/CFS/FM. Not that many people imported raw puffer fish in Upstate New York. In our outbreak of roughly 220 persons, I could not find any evidence of an enormous sushi party in Orleans County in 1985.

But what was fascinating was that this specific poisoning did cause symptoms that were essentially indistinguishable from the neuro-immune fatigue that follows a case of mononucleosis. The same holds true with the neurologic outcomes of persons with carbon monoxide poisoning, and possibly heavy metal poisoning. I have evaluated a patient with typical ME/CFS/FM following documented and clear-cut lead poisoning. Like carbon monoxide poisoning, the diagnosis is only known if the acute poisoning is detected accurately. These cases of neuro-immune fatigue are caused by neurologic injury.

But they also add another important element. What specifically causes the symptoms of heavy metal poisoning? The New York State Health Department recommends that pregnant women not eat any of the fish in our Great Lakes because of contamination with literally hundreds of neurotoxins. We know the site of injury in heavy metal poisoning; it is far down the chain of events in the energy production metabolic pathway. And, as we will discuss later, it is quite likely that a similar injury takes place in neuro-immune fatigue.

Organophosphate Poisoning

I don't know if it is appropriate to have a favorite poison, but organophosphates have always been close to my heart. In Upstate New York - home to Love Canal, the nuclear waste dump of West Valley, and the Niagara Falls chemical plants with its hundreds of superfund sites that will never be cleaned up, we have lots of toxins to boast. But the reason organophosphates are my favorite is these poisons are sprayed weekly over the orchards, and dumped from planes over the crop fields all summer long. On a nice spring day you breathe in a bucket of the pesticide when you drive by an orchard.

In the UK, vats of pesticides are made on farms and sheep are dipped in the vats to kill insects. Unlucky farmers who fall into sheep dip become ill with organophosphate poisoning, and have residual symptoms suggestive of Neuro-immune fatigue. Organophosphates were sprayed into the small tents of the Gulf War soldiers several times a day to kill the sand fleas, and the soldiers slept in the spray.

Organophosphates act as poisons to insects by blocking transmission of the neurotransmitter acetylcholine (ACh). Unfortunately for people, this neurotransmitter is important in humans as well. Investigators in the UK did an interesting study; they looked at persons with "chronic fatigue syndrome" without an obvious cause, and compared them to patients with Gulf War syndrome, and illness following organophosphate exposure (sheep dip). The three groups of patients all met diagnostic criteria for CFS, meaning that they had a similar pattern of symptoms. Of great interest is that there were differences in the acetylcholine tests. This represents the first study which could differentiate subgroups of persons with neuro-immune fatigue (Khan-2004).

Stress

There are two large groups of stress: physical stress and emotional stress. The latter has always been a sensitive topic to persons with

ME/CFS/FM because of fear that people will call them fruitcakes if the illness turns out to be caused by "stress." But stress is an important physiologic factor in the development of many illnesses and should not be ignored.

Most clinicians who study ME/CFS/FM have seen patients become ill during severe physical stress. I would guess that I have seen over thirty superbly trained athletes who developed the illness at the peak of physical abilities. One runner became acutely ill halfway through his twentieth marathon; one swimmer became ill during a very strenuous workout, and so on. It is possible that severe physical stress plays a role that has been poorly understood up until recently. Drs. Van Ness, Snell, and Staci Stevens have been looking into the possibility of over-training as a specific cause of neuro-immune fatigue. Again, this possibility helps to define the chain of events essential to the development of symptoms.

Emotional stress is also a possible cause, although when a person begins their illness nightmare with a nervous breakdown, it is rarely diagnosed as ME/CFS/FM. More frequently, the onset of the illness is clouded by the added emotional stresses of being unable to attend work, the resulting financial problems, and the confusion of the turbulent first six months. In this situation, emotional stresses are secondary to the onset of the illness rather than the cause of it. By the way, reducing emotional stress does improve the symptoms of neuro-immune fatigue by improving the ability to cope with the illness, not by a true reduction in symptom severity.

Conclusion

As time passes the list of causes of neuro-immune fatigue grows by leaps. Vitamin D deficiency, cancer chemotherapy, and silicone implants have been implicated. The body is enormously complex, but it does not have an infinite expression of symptoms. A headache is pain originating in the blood vessels of the brain. There may be five hundred different causes of the blood vessel reaction, but the headache is the same.

This is also true of neuro-immune fatigue. Like headache, it is defined by a shared pattern of symptoms. And it represents the end (symptomatic) expression of a series of events. We can now see that this series of events may be initiated by both infections and non-infectious insults. However, it is of greater importance to understand the resulting change in the metabolic pathways that permit these insults to express their debilitating symptoms.

## References

Ash-Bernal R, Wall C, Komaroff A, Bell D, Oas J, Payman R, et al. Vestibular function tests anomalies in patients with chronic fatigue syndrome. Acta Otolaryngol 1995;115:9-17

Bruno, RL. Paralytic versus non-paralytic polio": a distinction without a difference? Am J Phys Med Rehab. 1999; 79:4-12

Chaudhuri A, Behan P. Fatigue in neurological disorders. Lancet 2004;363(9413):978-988

Frohman E, Racke M, Raine C. Multiple Sclerosis - the plaque and its pathogenesis. NEJM 2006;354:942-955.

Khan F, Kennedy G, Spence V, Newton D, Belch J. Peripheral cholinergic function in humans with chronic fatigue syndrome, Gulf War syndrome and with illness following organophosphate exposure. Clin Sci 2004;106:183-189

Pearn J. Neurology of ciguatera. J Neurol Neurosurg Psychiatry. 2001; 70: 4-8

# Chapter 5: Genetic Influences

Genetic influences, also called host responses, are a critical factor in every illness. Ultimately, every biochemical reaction in our bodies is controlled or influenced by our genes. And, to a certain degree, the expression of nearly every illness is dependent upon our genes. As an example, if one hundred people were to contract poliovirus, only five of them would get paralytic polio. This is called the host response, the way in which a host responds to an infectious, physical, or toxic insult.

In neuro-immune fatigue, the host response is particularly important and has become a major part of the recent research. In my observations of the outbreak in Lyndonville, New York, there were 220 persons who developed chronic fatigue for more than six months. Most of these persons started with a flu-like infection, and there was a strong family incidence, implying either shared infectious agent, shared environmental factors or shared genetic influences. Interestingly, there were many persons who had what looked like the same initial infection causing profound fatigue for a month or two who never went on to develop the chronic fatigue. It is my assumption that these lucky persons did not have the host response or genetic factors that supported the illness. Some people got it, and some did not.

To illustrate the relationship of genetics to human experience I would like to summarize a study published recently about variations in a gene and the experience of pain (Diatchenko-05). In this study, the authors established a measure of pain sensitivity and then compared the degree of pain with several known variations (haplotypes) of a gene for an enzyme involved in neurotransmission. They were able to show that the severity of pain a person experienced was directly related to the variation of this particular gene. This is not a question of whether the person is or is not a wimp, implying either effective or non-effective coping methods; it is a biologic response beyond conscious control.

In ME/CFS/FM the degree of sensitivity to pain changes when a person develops the illness, so it is not purely a genetic predisposition. However, there is undoubtedly a genetic factor (or factors) but would permit the change in pain sensitivity. Ultimately, I would expect that this type of study will help in developing treatments for pain, which of course will help those with neuro-immune fatigue.

Twin studies in ME/CFS/FM

Clinicians seeing many patients with ME/CFS/FM have long been aware that it runs in families. In my own estimates I would guess that nearly 30% of persons with neuro-immune fatigue have at least one other immediate family member with a similar pattern of symptoms. This other family member may not have either the severity or number of symptoms to qualify as meeting various diagnostic criteria of ME/CFS/ FM, but the symptom pattern is not a coincidence, nor is it empathy.

There have been several twin studies looking at the presence of disabling fatigue and virtually all have shown an increase in the illness in twins, more in identical than in fraternal twins. This would imply that genetics plays a significant role, more than shared environment or shared infectious agents. In one study the prevalence for fatigue itself was 50% (Buchwald-01).

In one interesting study, 1,468 twin pairs were questioned for the presence of both disabling fatigue and depression. While the genetics can be daunting and the ability to measure fatigue and depression from questionnaires difficult, the models used suggested that both short duration fatigue and prolonged fatigue were familial. No gender differences were found. Furthermore, "for both short-duration fatigue and prolonged fatigue, the majority of the genetic and environmental influences variance is specific to disabling fatigue and distinct from depression. This suggests that fatigued states in children should be considered as valid entities in their own right and not as variants of depression." They also say that "unexplained disabling fatigue in childhood is substantially familial and has mainly an independent etiology from depression." (Fowler-06)

Formal Genetic Studies

There have been a number of genetic studies in ME/CFS/FM and it is a rapidly emerging field. In this section I will only superficially explore this area, as it is an extremely technical subject, still in its infancy. But several groups are doing wonderful studies including those of Stephen Kerr, Gow, Susan Vernon and others.

In the first chapter, mention was made of the Dubbo study in Australia. An attempt was made in that study to analyze the genetics (genomics) of those who developed neuro-immune fatigue after infectious mononucleosis and two other infections (Vernon-06). In this study, cells were evaluated for 3800 genes every few weeks for a year to evaluate for a pattern. What the researchers found was that the gene transcription patterns after an infection with Epstein-Barr virus was different between those who recovered normally and those who developed ME/CFS/FM. The authors stated, "We found that individuals who suffered from post-infective fatigue had a distinct gene expression profile during the acute illness compared to those whose illness resolved. Evaluation of the gene expression profile over the course of the year implicated an altered host response to EBV and mitochondrial dysfunction in those who developed post-infective fatigue."

The implications of this are profound. It suggests that during the first week of infectious mononucleosis, it could be possible to tell which persons will go on to develop neuro-immune fatigue. And if this were true, then it could be possible to identify the exact defects responsible, perhaps even correct them prior to developing the illness.

Diagnostic Tests

Studies are accumulating which will allow a diagnostic test based on gene expression to identify patients with ME/CFS/FM from healthy persons. And eventually these gene expression markers will identify specific subtypes of the illness. In an old and small study, Susan Vernon extracted the RNA from cells of five patients with neuro-immune fatigue and compared it to the genes of seventeen healthy persons. Eight different genes, several related to immune function were differentially expressed and could separate cases from controls (Vernon-02).

Jonathon Kerr's group in London has done a similar study using different genes. They were able to show differential expression in thirty-five genes. When these were confirmed with PCR technology, fifteen genes were upregulated compared to normal; one was down-regulated. The genes profile suggests T cell activation and abnormal nerve and mitochondrial function (Kaushik-05).

It is too early to go to your health care provider and ask for a gene test to diagnose neuro-immune fatigue. But it may not be that far away.

Conclusion

It has been many years since ME/CFS/FM began to be the subject of serious scrutiny. Clinicians have described the signs and symptoms of this illness since the early outbreaks: Gilliam in 1938 described the Los Angeles Hospital outbreak, Sigurdsson described the Iceland epidemic of 1949, and Ramsey described the Royal Free Hospital outbreak of 1950.

But in these days of "managed" medical care reduced to formulas that can be practiced by eight-year-olds, no one listens. The old fashioned scientific approach does not work to help people's suffering anymore. I guess it can be argued it did not work that well in the old days, either.

But a new science is coming to life, evolving from the rituals of health insurance company medicine. This new science can measure specific genetic material and signals, detect which genes are active or inactive (gene expression), and how these genes communicate with each other and to different parts of the cell. This new approach marks a major break from traditional medicine as it begins to look past organ-specific diagnoses and search diagnoses at a molecular level. More importantly, it holds the promise of treatments inconceivable in years past: how to induce, or turn on or off specific genes active in specific diseases. Brave new world.

## References

Buchwald D, Herrell R, Ashton S, et al. A twin study of chronic fatigue. Psychosom Med. 2001; 63:936-943

Diatchenko L, Slade G, Nackley A, et al. Genetic basis for individual variation in pain perception and the development of a chronic condition. Hum Mol Genet 2005;14(1):135-143

Fowler T, Rice F, Thapar A, Farmer A. Relationship between disabling fatigue and depression in children. British Journal of Psychiatry 2006;189:247-253

Furberg H, Olarte M, Afari N, Goldberg J, Buchwald D, Sullivan P. The prevalence of self-reported chronic fatigue in a U.S. twin registry. J Psychosom Res 2005;59(5):283-290

Kaushik N, Fear D, Richards S, McDermott C, Nuwaysir E, Kellam P, et al. Gene expression in peripheral blood mononuclear cells from patients with chronic fatigue syndrome. Journal of Clinical Pathology. 2005;(8)

Vernon S, Whistler T, Cameron B, Hickie I, Reeves W, Lloyd A. Preliminary evidence of mitochondrial dysfunction associated with post-infectious fatigue after acute infection with Epstein-Barr virus. BMC Infectious Diseases 2006;6: http://www.biomedcentral.com/1471-2334/1476/1416

Vernon S, Unger E, Dimulescu I, Rajeevan M, Reeves W. Utility of the blood for gene expression profiling and biomarker discovery in chronic fatigue syndrome. Disease Markers 2002;18(4):193-199

# Chapter 6: The Immune-Cytokine Cascade

Many, many years ago when I was in medical school one of the hardest subjects to study was the blood clotting cascade in hematology.

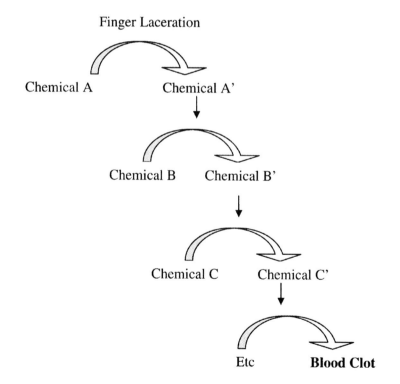

The cascade looked like a series of water fountains. The one at the very top (Chemical A becomes A') causes a change in chemical B to make it B'; that causes chemical C to become C', and so on for twenty-five or thirty steps. Each step had its own rules and enzymes and was influenced by different factors. It was impossible to memorize, particularly so because not all the steps were known at that time.

Unfortunately for me, the body seems to love cascades. Moreover, we do not understand the specific waterfall steps of the immune system cascade perfectly. Add to that, each step can go in different directions – the immune system talks to the nervous system, and the nervous system regulates the endocrine system, and so on. But the cascade creates a redundancy or safety net which makes it less disasterous if something goes wrong.

And of course, with every step something can go wrong. In the blood clotting cascade, if one enzyme or protein is missing the result is hemophilia A. With another error it is delta granule storage disease; another is Von Willebrand's disease. They may look similar from the symptoms – a cut does not stop bleeding – but the mechanism that has gone wrong in the cascade is different in each illness. In neuro-immune fatigue there is a problem, or problems, with the immune activation cascade. The end result of this problem or these problems is the symptom complex of ME/CFS/FM.

In the first chapter of this section we discussed the evidence pointing to certain infections causing ME/CFS/FM. The next question is how do these infections cause the prolonged symptoms, and for some, the flu that never ends. The answer to this question involves the immune mechanism set off by the infection, and specifically the abnormal immune mechanism that allows for persistence of symptoms even after the obvious infection has gone away.

In the second chapter we discussed the non-infectious causes, and that there is a variation from the cascade initiated by standard infections. Yet many of the same cytokines are involved, and ultimately the cascades which result in neuro-immune fatigue come to a common point.

It appears that this common point where the cascades merge is in the area of cellular metabolism, more specifically the inability of converting oxygen into energy, or cellular hypoxia. In this chapter we will be looking primarily at the immune mechanism (or abnormal immune mechanism) following an infectious insult; we will be ignoring the neuro-immune fatigue caused by toxic exposure, brain injury, heavy metal poisoning, cigatura poisoning, and the like as it is likely that each cascade will be slightly different. Rather than identify specific steps, we will concentrate on the concept of the neuro-immune cytokine cascade.

In the early days of ME/CFS/FM research in the US, emphasis rested upon looking at the Epstein-Barr virus as the cause to the immune activation that seemed to be the hallmark of the illness. The name Chronic Fatigue Immune Dysfunction Syndrome (CFIDS) dates from this time and remains accurate as a name for some types of this illness. However, most patients assumed that this meant that patients with ME/CFS/FM had an "under-active" immune illness response, an immune deficiency. The dominent aspect is just the opposite, an over-active immune state. Neuro-immune fatigue is a condition where the immune system is spinning its tires in the sand, getting really tired and going nowhere.

There are immune deficiencies in neuro-immune fatigue, which some scientist/clinicians like Dr. Nancy Klimas and Dr. Roberto Patarca have been studying for years. The natural killer cells are off both in number and function, and some cellular immune responses are delayed. Arguments rage in the literature about the usefulness of these studies because they may relate to specific subgroups. The immune deficiencies may be the critical issue if they turn out to cause persistent infection and the resulting immune over-reaction. For now, let us turn our attention to the cytokine cascade activated by the initiating infection.

Definitions

For the rookies among the readers, there are a few basic definitions that must be mastered before proceeding. Cytokines are chemicals made by the cell which act to carry out essential functions. While there are many subgroups (perhaps thousands) of these messaging chemicals, I will oversimplify by referring to them collectively as cytokines. The ones I will be discussing are related primarily to immune function and communication between the brain and the immune systems. The group of cytokines that seems to play the biggest role are the "pro-inflammatory" cytokines.

One cytokine that we will be referring to extensively in the next chapters is interferon, and there are three major types established so far: α, β, and γ (alpha, beta, and gamma). This is one of the first cytokines discovered, and as I recall from the history, it was named because when someone had a viral infection, a chemical was produced by the immune system that "interfered" and prevented another virus from causing an infection at the same time. The good news is that you only get one virus at a time; the bad news is that interferon makes you feel really sick. It has been studied extensively and has been used to treat illnesses such as cancer, hepatitis and multiple sclerosis.

Another cytokine is TNF, (tumor necrosis factor) and it also comes in various Greek subgroups. It is used to treat rheumatoid arthritis, psoriasis, and other illnesses. The interleukins are cytokines that act as communicators in an unbelieveably complex cellular system. There are thousands of tasks to do within the cell and every task requires a specific mechanism to carry it out.

Getting the Flu

With an infection, the body jumps into action to defend itself, but usually not for several days. For example, if you are in the checkout lane at the grocery store and the person next to you coughs on you, you breathe in the flu virus. The virus particle lodges in your airway and begins to multiply; yet you feel just fine. In fact you feel fine for three days or so (the incubation period) even though the virus is growing like mad. Then, Saturday afternoon, at exactly three PM, you come down with the flu: fever, headache, aches and pains, exhaustion, sore throat, nausea..... What actually happened on Saturday was that your body recognized the attack by the flu virus and began making cytokines to begin the counter-attack. And the cytokines make you feel sick.

You stay in bed for a few days while the battle rages. The battle is carried out on several fronts and after the immune system makes antibodies the infection is brought under control. When that happens the production of cytokines slows down, stops, and you feel better. A few more days and you are back to normal, if everything goes right.

The production of these cytokines, (specifically interferon, IL-1, IL-6, and TNF) is known to cause the symptoms of illness, often called "acute sickness behavior." This term does not imply that there is anything artificial or psychological about the behavior, it is as real as limping behavior in a person with a broken leg. These effects of cytokines were discovered during trials where the cytokines were given to healthy volunteers who then developed fever and other symptoms.

In neuro-immune fatigue something goes wrong. The infection may be an ordinary "garden variety" virus, an enterovirus, or the Epstein-Barr virus of mononucleosis. But in a person with the genetic vulnerability the process does not shut down and the flu-like symptoms persist for months, years, sometimes for the rest of his or her life. It is this abnormal mechanism that is our center of attention.

The symptoms caused by cytokines differ from "end organ" symptoms. For example, weakness is a common symptom in ME/CFS/FM, but muscle testing with electrodes does not indicate muscle fiber disease. Characteristically, the sensation of profound weakness is experienced by those persons given cytokine injections despite normal muscles. Confusion and problems with memory and attention are symptoms caused by cytokines and in experimental subjects, when the cytokine wears off these cognitive symptoms resolve without damage to brain cells (presumably). It is precisely because these symptoms are not caused by diseases of muscle or joint that medical providers have ignored them. If you go to the doctor with a cough caused by the flu you are patted on the head and ignored, unless you cough up gobs of lung tissue. Then it is taken a little more seriously.

Examples of the Cytokine Cascade or Cytokine Storm

Among the many frustrations of seeing the reality and the importance of neuro-immune fatigue questioned over the past twenty years is that there are well known examples of cytokines causing serious illness.

One interesting study looked at the relationship between pro-inflammatory cytokines and the degree of fatigue in patients with multiple sclerosis (MS). Those MS patients without significant fatigue had much lower levels of pro-inflammatory cytokines. This study is of value as there is known to be a substantial variation in the degree in fatigue in patients with MS (Heesen-06)

A published example of a cytokine storm occurred in healthy volunteers given an experimental drug (Sunthralingam-06). The drug was an antibody whose function was to stimulate T cells, which, it turns out, it did too well. The subjects were healthy volunteers and the drug caused a cytokine cascade involving many different cytokines, including tumor necrosis factor alpha, gamma interferon and several interleukins. The healthy volunteers all became very ill and had to be admitted to an intensive care unit. The importance of this disasterous trial was to show the progression of a cytokine storm precipitated by a specific monoclonal antibody in previously healthy persons. In medical school I used to volunteer for these kinds of trials because I was broke.

There are many different cytokine cascades. Variations in ME/ CFS/FM may relate to variations in individual cascades, which are just now beginning to be studied. But the essential point has been established. Cytokine cascades cause symptoms and illness. Sometimes the illnesses caused are very severe, even fatal. It remains to be seen what will be the exact profile or profiles that comprise what we have been up to now calling ME/CFS/FM.

## Cytokine Production in Neuro-immune Fatigue

Over the past ten years there has been a concerted attempt to measure the cytokine response in ME/CFS/FM. Unfortunately it is not a simple process. The blood stream, where the medical tests get done, is far away from the cellular mechanisms. It is generally agreed that an abnormal response exists, with the normal balance between pro-inflammatory cytokines and the cellular responses being disrupted. In the studies mentioned earlier by Dr. Kerr and associates, TNF-$\alpha$ and IFN-$\gamma$ are present for long periods of time when parvovirus initiates ME/CFS/FM. They were even able to demonstrate an abnormal TNF-$\alpha$ gene which could affect the development of persistent fatigue.

In one interesting study, the cytokine IL-6 was injected into patients and healthy controls as it is known to cause a pattern of symptoms very similar to neuro-immune fatigue. As expected the cytokine caused an increase in fatigue, headache, muscle and joint pain. Other studies have looked at cytokines in the spinal fluid and during stress responses.

One question that has not been resolved is whether the cytokine cascade of ME/CFS/FM is due to ongoing infection, or if it is abnormal despite no measurable infection present. It is a chicken and egg question, and at present there is no clear answer. It is likely that when the research answers are in, it will be both. There will be an element of ongoing infection due to an abnormal cytokine cascade.

2'-5' A Synthetase and Rnase L

This the next step in the process was started by research by Robert Suhadolnik and his group around 1995 and continues actively at the present time. An enzyme called 2'-5'A Synthetase is normally stimulated by the cytokine interferon to make RNase L, an enzyme that can "chew up" viral RNA. Therefore it is part of the normal anti-viral defense system. In neuro-immune fatigue there is a glitch present with an abnormal protein present (the 37kDa fragment) in those most severely affected by the illness.

There are three ways that an abnormality in this system may cause problems in neuro-immune fatigue. First it allows for the continuous stimulation and production of interferon which, as we will see, could be a major player in the symptoms of the illness. Secondly, it may permit the persistence of the initiating infection. And thirdly, an excess of RNase L can cause other difficulties down the road, because its actions are not limited to viral RNA. It may be chewing up good RNA as well. In a follow-up study it was noted that 72% of patients had an excess of the abnormal protein in ME/CFS/FM while only 1% of the normal population had it.

Hepatitis C Study

In 2004 a remarkable study was presented at the IACFS scientific meetings that began to draw together this information. So far we have seen that the immune system is overactive or "upregulated" in neuro-immune fatigue, and we know that people feel lousy, but are the two facts connected? Does the presence of these cytokines actually cause the persistence of symptoms?

Interferon is a cytokine used as an anti-viral treatment in certain illnesses such as Hepatitis C. In a study conducted by Dr. Charles Raison, patients with known Hepatitis C were given interferon. Prior to treatment 22% of the patients had significant chronic fatigue and 3% would fit specific criteria for chronic fatigue syndrome. After treatment with interferon 70% of the subjects had chronic fatigue and 30% met criteria. What this means is that administration of the cytokine interferon transformed some persons with a known persistent virus (Hepatitis C) but without chronic fatigue into having ME/CFS/FM along with their hepatitis C. The importance of this study should not be overlooked. We finally have a model for the progression of the illness that can be studied, and, with any good luck, treatment interventions can be tested.

Autoimmunity

Many persons with ME/CFS/FM have some autoimmunity. It has never been clear whether this autoimmunity is another spin off (epiphenomenon) of the abnormal over-active immune response, or whether it is important to the generation of symptoms. Up to 25% of neuro-immune fatigue patients have an abnormal ANA, a test that can suggest the disease lupus erythematosis. The more you look for autoantibodies, the more of them can be found, but it is unlikely that these autoantibodies are doing much harm.

Because the immune system is "revved-up", it is looking for something to attack. When this happens it can sometimes attack normal tissue, causing autoimmunity. This is similar to allergies where the immune response is directed toward otherwise harmless pollen or cat dander.

In true autoimmune disease demonstrable tissue damage can be found, as in rheumatoid arthritis. An interesting concept is the possibility that multiple sclerosis is neuro-immune fatigue with overlying brain tissue autoimmunity due to an injury of the blood-brain barrier (Heesen-06). To a carpenter everything looks like a nail.

Finally, a word about medications that increase serotonin, commonly known as "antidepressants." It is known that blockade of at least one serotonin receptor will reduce several cytokines including tumor necrosis factor, and some of the interleukins. Reduction in pain for some persons with ME/CFS/FM may be a side effect of these medications, and not due to the "antidepressant" effects.

In a standard infection like the flu, we can see that the viral infection and the stimulated cytokines cause symptoms, but we never paid any attention because in a few days the cytokine cascade shuts down and the symptoms go away. Who cares why the cytokines cause exhaustion, headache, muscle and joint pain? But with neuro-immune fatigue the process does not stop, so the next step becomes critical: how does this cytokine cascade cause symptoms? If we can understand the answer to this question we will be able to understand how to intervene and stop the symptoms.

Conclusions

There are several conclusions to be drawn:

1) Persons with ME/CFS/FM have persistent immune activation as if there were a persistent infection going on. More technically, there is an abnormal shift of the immune response to Th2 instead of the normal balance between Th1 and Th2.
2) There is a persistence of cytokine secretion that is likely responsible for the persistence of symptoms.
3) The symptoms of neuro-immune fatigue can be temporarily reproduced by injections of cytokines such as interferon and interleukins.
4) Neuro-immune fatigue can be caused by treating a patient with hepatitis C with interferon.

References

Arnold M, Papanicolaou D, O'Grady J, Lotsikas A, Dale J, Straus S, et al. Using an interleukin-6 challenge to evaluate neuropsychological performance in chronic fatigue syndrome. Psychol Med 2002;32:1075-1089.

Dantzer R. Cytokine-induced sickness behavior: Where do we stand? Brain, Behavior, and Immunity 2001;15:7-24

De Meirleir K, Bisbal C, Campine I, De Becker P, Salezada T, Demettre E, LeBleu B. A 37kDa 2-5A binding protein as a potential biochemical marker for chronic fatigue syndrome. Am J Med. 2000; 108:99-105.

Gaab J, Rohleder N, Heitz V, Engert V, Schad T, Schurmeyer T, et al. Stress-induced changes in LPS-induced pro-inflammatory cytokine production in chronic fatigue syndrome. Psychoneuroendocrinology 2005;30:188-198.

Sharara AI, Perkins DJ, Misukonis MA, Chan SU, Dominitz JA Weinberg JB 1997 Interferon (IFN)-alpha activation of human blood mononuclear cells in vitro and in vivo for nitric oxide synthetase (NOS) type 2 mRNA and protein expression: possible relationship of induced NOS2 to the anti-hepatitis C effects of IFN-alpha in vivo. 1997. J Exp Med. 186:1495-1502.

Gerrity T, Papanicolaou D, Amsterdam J, Bingham S, Grossman A, Hedrick T, et al. Immunologic Aspects of chronic fatigue syndrome. Neuroimmunomodulation 2004;11:351-357.

Heesen C, Nawrath L, Reich C, Bauer N, Schulz K, Gold S. Fatigue in multiple sclerosis: an example of cytokine mediated sickness behaviour? J Neurol Neurosurg Psychiatry 2006;77:34-39

Kaushik N, Fear D, Richards S, McDermott C, Nuwaysir E, Kellam P, et al. Gene expression in peripheral blood mononuclear cells from patients with chronic fatigue syndrome. Journal of Clinical Pathology (8)

Kerr J, McCoy M, Burke B, Matteyt D, Pravica V, Hutchinson I. Cytokine gene polymorphisms associated with symptomatic parvovirus B19 infection. J Clin Path 2003;56:725-727.

Raison C, Borisov A, Broadwell SD, Capuron L, Woolwine B, Nemeroff C, et al. Syndrome of chronic fatigue in patients receiving interferon-alpha for chronic hepatitis C virus infection. Presented at the 2004 AACFS Meetings, Madison, Wisc 10/9/04 2004.

Suhadolnik RJ, Peterson DL, O'Brien K, Cheney PR, Herst CV, Reichenbach NL, Kron N, Horvath SE, Iacono, KT, Adelson ME, DeMeirleir K, DeBecker P, Charubala R, Wolfgang P. Biochemical evidence for a novel low molecular weight 2-5Adependent Rnase L in chronic fatigue syndrome. Journal of Interferon and Cytokine Research. 1997; 7:377-385.

Sunthralingam G, Perry M, Ward S, SJ B, Castello-Cortes A, MD B, et al. Cytokine storm in a phase 1 trial of the anti-CD28 Monoclonal antibody TGN1412. NEJM 2006;355(10):1018-1028

Tomoda A, Joudoi T, Rabab E, Matsumoto T, Park T, Miike T. Cytokine production and modulation: comparison of patients with chronic fatigue syndrome and normal controls. Psychiatry Research. 2005;134:101-104

Vollmer-Conna U. Acute sickness behavior: an immune system-to-brain communication? Psychol Med 01;31:761-767

Warren G, McKendrick M, Peet M. The role of essential fatty acids in chronic fatigue syndrome.

# Chapter 7: The Role of Nitric Oxide Metabolism

Now comes the difficult part. For those of you out there who are rookies, fasten your seat belts. As mentioned before what I will be attempting to discuss in this chapter is not new, it has been discussed by Drs. Martin Pall, Paul Cheney, Kenny DeMerlier and several others whom I consider my teachers. But while it is not necessarily brand new, it is daunting to say the least, and for that readon is not familiar to many. So buckle up rookies, here we go.

It is time to approach the mechanism that translates infection or nervous system injury and its subsequent abnormal immune and metabolic response into the symptoms of neuro-immune fatigue. It is time for the brave and courageous to step forward. We have come to a critical junction in the road where causes evolve to consequences, where initiating events converge into a metabolic prism and emerge as a rainbow of unpleasant symptoms.

A word about the human body: so far, we have been talking about mechanisms going wrong, immune systems stuck in fifth gear, resulting in pain and suffering. It would seem that God really messed up here with major design flaws. The reason that God stays hidden from us most of the time is that He would have a whole lot of lawsuits to deal with, or that He is really tired of human whining.

Actually, I marvel at the complexity of the human body. The fact that it works at all, even some of the time, is truly amazing. When I study cellular mechanisms uncovered by today's science, I feel like an astronomer looking into the nighttime sky filled with five hundred billion galaxies, each with five hundred billion stars. And those are just the ones our telescopes can see. Each galaxy and each star is immeasurably complex, ultimately made of atoms and spinning electrons. It gets complicated when you add in quantum mechanics.

When illness occurs we should do everything in our power to search its cause and find remedies. Science is man's feeble attempt to do that and it has been successful in some illnesses. Compared to the incredible subtlety and sophistication of the body's workings, man's understanding is slight indeed.

But enough of philosophy. Back to business.

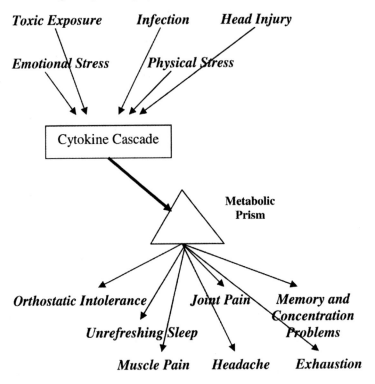

## The Prism

It is the premise of this monograph that the ME/CFS/FM junction box where cause or causes become consequence is discreet and concrete, not some vague psychic or psychological mechanism. And because it is a discreet, physiologic mechanism, it has the potential to be studied, altered, manipulated, and possibly corrected when it goes haywire, just like any other physiologic mechanism in the body. This prism or junction box in the neuro-immune fatigue spectrum of illnesses is nitric oxide metabolism.

The symptoms of ME/CFS/FM come directly by alterations in the production, concentration, or elimination of nitric oxide. As we will describe in more detail in the rest of this book, there are three groups of ME/CFS/FM symptoms: fatigue, pain and blood flow. Two of these symptom groups (vasculopathy and central sensitization) stem from the direct action of nitric oxide on body tissues. These two symptom groups are annoying and unpleasant, but do not result in the activity limitation (fatigue) of the illness, the most disabling symptom. The third group of symptoms is the result of impaired energy production by nitric oxide itself or oxidative damage by its toxic by-products superoxide and peroxynitrite. This third group of symptoms – impaired energy production through impaired oxidative phosphorylation – is the primary cause of the disability of ME/CFS/FM.

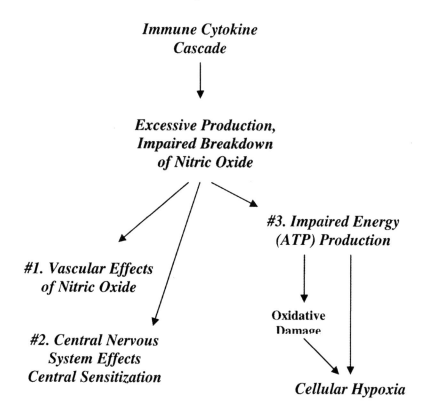

Nitric Oxide

Nitric oxide is a remarkable substance. By the way, it is not "nitrous oxide," the laughing gas in the dentist's office. Nitric oxide, abbreviated as NO, is a tiny, evanescent gas that takes part in nearly all cellular processes. It is so short lived that it is not possible to measure accurately, which has been one of the biggest reasons it has remained hidden all these years. It was not even discovered until the 1980s, and with some sort of dubious honor, it was called the "molecule of the year." Nitric oxide is not to be thought of as a bad guy or evil; it is essential to life. But like all other substances existing in the human body, it must exist in the correct concentrations.

Nitric oxide's first and probably main claim to fame has been its role in the cardiovascular system. For the past twenty years it has been studied intensely because of its importance in cardiovascular health. It is a vasodilator, relaxing the muscles that surround blood vessels, thus allowing more blood to pass. When someone is having chest pain from angina or a heart attack, they are given nitroglycerine which dilates the blood vessels to the heart and reduces the chest pain. Nitroglycerine also inhibits platelet activation, thus limiting the size of a heart attack.

Nitric oxide has many diverse functions. It is a neurotransmitter with an important role in pain perception, modifies cytotoxicity and immunity, stimulates cellular adhesion, and helps regulate apoptosis or programmed cell death. It lowers blood pressure by dilating blood vessels. Nitric oxide stimulates the release of noradrenalin.

Like any fundamental cellular substance there are lots of potential problems. When too much is produced, it will lower blood pressure excessively, even causing cardiovascular shock in some instances. And its breakdown produces two toxic products, superoxide and peroxynitrite, toxic metabolites that have been recognized and studied for years. They are the the target of most anti-oxidants advertised to cure everything from heart disease to old age. But the system is complex, and a little vitamin C is not enough to correct ME/CFS/FM.

Production of Nitric Oxide

Nitric oxide is produced from the amino acid l-arginine by the enzyme nitric oxide synthetase (NOS). There are four forms of this enzyme discovered so far, the inducible NOS (iNOS), endothelial NOS (eNOS), neuronal NOS (nNOS), and mitochondrial NOS, (mtNOS). Each is slightly different, but one that stands out for hypothetical reasons in the iNOS. This is because infection induces the formation of nitric oxide. Presumably this is advantageous because the resulting nitric oxide will dilate blood vessels and increase blood flow to an infected area, thus helping fight the infection.

The induction of nitric oxide by infection makes good theoretical sense in ME/CFS/FM because of the connection to infection and the cytokine cascade discussed earlier. But nitric oxide is also produced in neurologic injury. In fact, it is likely that the majority of damage following a stroke is due to the toxic nitric oxide by-products. With head trauma, brain swelling reduces blood flow to neuronal tissue, and the resulting damage is mediated in part by nitric oxide and its by-products. With increased understanding of nNOS and iNOS, major gains are likely in the treatment of neurologic disease.

I should resist the temptation to diverge into endless side discussions, but I cannot resist here. There is an animal model of multiple sclerosis (MS) which looks and acts just like MS in furry little rodents. It is very useful for us to study MS and get hints for possible treatments, although it is not great if you happen to be a laboratory rat. In this model, it appears that nitric oxide and its by-product peroxynitrite disrupt the blood brain barrier allowing the formation of autoantibodies to myelin. In this animal model, MS can be prevented by drugs that inhibit iNOS and scavenge the excess nitric oxide (Hooper-97). This implies that nitric oxide is at the root of multiple sclerosis, another possible reason why the symptoms are so similar to neuro-immune fatigue.

Septic Shock

A good place to start the discussion of the role of nitric oxide in ME/CFS/FM is a discussion of septic shock. Septic shock is a well known, often fatal, condition that occurs as a consequence of bacterial infection. In its most typical presentation, an elderly person develops a kidney infection and does not seek treatment early. The bacteria causing the kidney infection get into the blood stream and stimulate the enzyme iNOS. This causes a massive production of nitric oxide and the blood vessels dilate. When this happens the blood pressure falls and the person goes into cardiovascular shock. In the early stages of this process, treating the infection and blood pressure can reverse the damage, but left untreated it is fatal.

However, there is an interesting and critical next step. Sometimes even with good fluid and blood pressure treatment the condition is fatal. Death is not caused by the reduced blood flow to organs; it is the action of nitric oxide and its by-products poisoning the mitochondria. In 1997, Mitchell Fink used the expression "cytopathic hypoxia" to describe this reduction of oxygen consumption by tissues in sepsis. He called this "cytopathic hypoxia" because the problem was not due to lack of oxygen in the blood stream or tissues. It was an acquired defect in cellular respiration, the ability of the mitochondria to transform oxygen into energy.

The parallels with neuro-immune fatigue are striking. ME/CFS/FM is rarely, if ever, fatal, so persons with ME/CFS/FM should not panic. But usually an infection sets off the cytokine cascade, although on a much reduced scale from septic shock. Both septic shock and neuro-immune fatigue have blood flow abnormalities and reduced tissue energy generation. It is known that certain types of infection are more likely to produce excess nitric oxide, and ME/CFS/FM is more common following certain types of infection. As mentioned in the chapter on the cytokine cascade, interferon can cause ME/CFS/FM, and it is known that mononuclear cells of patients with hepatitis C have very little mRNA for the enzyme iNOS. However, as soon as they are treated with α interferon alpha, the iNOS enzyme is produced along with nitric oxide (Sharara-97).

Here I must restrain myself again from diving into hundreds of details relating to the possible relationship between nitric oxide and the symptoms of neuro-immune fatigue. The problem of a clinician dabbling in basic science is the lack of perspective and judgment that is gained by spending a lifetime studying a subject. But forgive me for being excited. The common denominator just may turn out to be chronically overproduced nitric oxide or a defect in the ability of the body to safely get rid of its breakdown products. It is just possible that ME/CFS/FM is a mild, but chronic, septic shock.

If you, gentle reader, have made it this far you are to be commended for your patience. The concepts of cellular medicine are difficult and represent a paradigm shift in medicine. It is no longer possible to classify an illness by organ systems only, and ME/CFS/FM is likely to lead the way in bringing this shift about. The good news is that it opens up whole new vistas of treatment possibilities.

But before you relax too much, let us discuss the symptom clusters. Chapter 8 will attempt to look at the vascular changes and Chapter 9 the abnormalities in the central nervous system that causes the excessive perception of sensory stimuli. In Chapter 10 we will look at the effects of defective nitric oxide breakdown and how that impairs energy production.

Conclusions

Neuro-immune fatigue is an illness with diverse and hard to define symptoms. It is possible to divide the various symptoms into three broad groups. The first is a "vasculopathy", abnormal dilation and contraction of the blood vessels which contribute to orthostatic intolerance, exhaustion, cognitive disturbance, pallor, headache, and other symptoms. The second group is "central sensitization", an abnormal sensitivity to sensory input, which contributes to the muscle and joint pain, headache, light and noise sensitivity, and chemical sensitivities. The third group (and perhaps the most important) is cellular hypoxia, the disruption of energy production in the mitochondria.

It is possible to hypothesize that all three of these groups of symptoms can follow from abnormalities in the nitric oxide metabolic pathway. An excess nitric oxide may be responsible for the vasculopathy and central sensitization. But the most damage would be done by excessive production of nitric oxide by products, peroxynitrite and superoxide. These toxic by-products interfere with energy production in the mitochondria by inhibiting oxidative phosphorylation.

Neuro-immune fatigue is a spectrum of related disorders: myalgic encephalopathy, chronic fatigue syndrome, orthostatic intolerance, fibromyalgia, and chemical sensitivities. The variation in symptom expression within each of these disorders, and from one part of the spectrum to another can be explained by the many steps that exist between the immune response following an infection and the prouction of energy by mitochondria. The illness variations most likely result from individual abnormalities in the specific steps of these metabolic cascades.

References

Fink M: Cytopathic hypoxia in sepsis. *Acta Anaesthesiol Scand* 1997, 41(Suppl 100):87-95.

Fink M: Bench-to-bedside review: Cytopathic hypoxia. *Critical Care* 2002, 6:491-499

Nijs J, Van de Velde B, De Meirleir K. Pain in patients with chronic fatigue syndrome: does nitric oxide trigger central central sentisization? Med Hypothesis. 2005; 64(3):558-62.

Hooper D, Bagastra O, Marini J, Zborek A, Ohnis S, Champion J, et al. Prevention of experimental allergic encephalomyelitis by targeting nitric oxide and peroxynitrite: Implications for the treatment of multiple sclerosis. PNAS 1997;94(6):2528-2533

Hooper D, Scott G, Zborek A, Mikheeva T, Kean, RB, Koprowski H, et al. Uric Acid, a peroxynitrite scavenger, inhibits CNAS inflammation, blood-CNS barrier permeability changes, and tissue damage in a mouse model of multiple sclerosis. The FASEB Journal 2000;14:691-698

Mayer B, ed. Nitric Oxide Handbook of Experimental Pharmacology Volume 143, Springer, NY 2000

Sharara AI, Perkins DJ, Misukonis MA, Chan SU, Dominitz JA Weinberg JB 1997 Interferon (IFN)-alpha activation of human blood mononuclear cells in vitro and in vivo for nitric oxide synthetase (NOS) type 2 mRNA and protein expression: possible relationship of induced NOS2 to the anti-hepatitis C effects of IFN-alpha in vivo. 1997. J Exp Med. 186:1495-1502.

# Chapter 8: Symptom Cluster #1: Vasculopathy

Vasculopathy is an awkward word. I don't like it very much. Vasculitis is much nicer, meaning inflammation of the blood vessels. A typical vasculitis doesn't occur in ME/CFS, but the word is clean, nice - it commands respect. Vasculopathy means that the vascular system (blood vessels) don't work very well. The term does not command respect. Then again, not much about neuro-immune fatigue commands respect. It is a disease localized in the basement of cellular function and gets expressed in nearly all organs. It is a disease of cellular metabolism, not of organ function.

However the ME/CFS/FM spectrum has a unique signature. It has signs and symptoms that differentiate it from all other clinical illnesses. Reluctance to accept, or even recognize this signature stems from the fact that these symptoms do not all originate from a single tissue, hormone, or organ. But they actually do fit a pattern that makes sense, and I would define this pattern by dividing the symptoms into three groups. The groups follow from the immune and metabolic cascade we have been attempting to describe, a cascade where nitric oxide and its effect upon mitochondrial function becomes critical.

One difficulty we will be exploring is that there is exists an overlap with more than one symptom group causing a specific symptom. Fatigue is the prime example. We will be relating fatigue, exhaustion, and activity limitation primarily to a reduction in cellular energy production (symptom cluster 3), but orthostatic intolerance related to blood vessel problems causes fatigue in its own right. Therefore, from a theoretical point of view with treatment in mind, all three of these symptom groups need to be treated at the same time. Let us start with the vasculopathy.

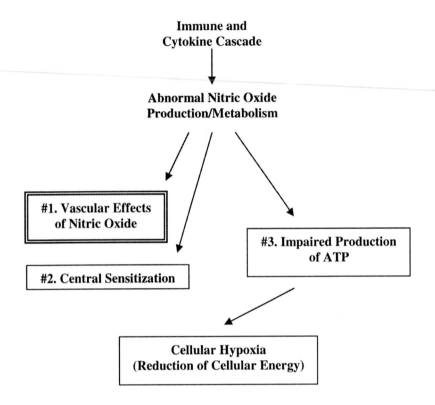

## Symptoms

In 1985 when ME/CFSFM was first coming to our attention, the vasculopathy was the first feature we noticed in our office. It started with a teenager who I saw in town walking along the sidewalk. He was a regular patient of mine and was well except that he had a flushing rash on his cheeks. His cheeks were bright red as he walked by and we greeted each other. Two days later he came into the office with a flu-like illness and his ordeal with ME/CFS/FM had begun.

In our first attempt to create diagnostic criteria for what we were witnessing we called this a rash which was not correct. It was flushing – dilated blood vessels of the cheeks that would alternate with pallor, a sickly pale color. And we observed others where this flushing occurred even before the malaise and fever. Perhaps the illness which set off our town's little adventure was parvovirus.

Regardless of the cause in retrospect, a change in blood vessel function is part of the symptom pattern of the illness. In the early days of neuro-immune fatigue research the blood vessel problems were felt to be due to abnormalities within the autonomic nervous system, and to this day, that continues to be argued. Are the blood vessels reacting differently because of excessive vasodilator tone due to nitric oxide or because of the autonomic nervous system? Unfortunately for those of us who would like a simple and clean answer, the two possibilities are connected.

Among the thousand names given to this illness, many describe the vasculopathy as primary: orthostatic intolerance, postural tachycardia, neurally mediated hypotension, delayed orthostatic hypotension, and so on. For the sake of simplicity I will lump these together as orthostatic intolerance, the inability to tolerate the upright position. Central to the symptoms of ME/CFS/FM is the fatigue, near-fainting sensation (pre-syncope), lightheadedness, dizziness, and cognitive problems of orthostatic intolerance. Headache is another important vascular symptom. It can be caused by the blood vessels being either too dilated or too constricted, both of which occur in migraine.

An interesting possibility is that the abnormalities in the hypothalamic-pituitary-adrenal axis (HPA axis) could be secondary to a vasculopathy. If there is abnormal blood flow to the brain, it is likely to affect the production of neuro-hormones. Researchers have historically been looking for been a "fixed" or mechanical problem to explain abnormalities in the production of growth hormone, cortisol, antidiuretic hormone and other neuro-hormones. But because there is no fixed injury like a brain tumor or stroke, endocrinologists have given up looking in frustration. The HPA axis variations in neuro-immune fatigue are not the central cause of the symptom pattern. And because they are an epiphenomenon of the vasculopathy, treating the illness with various hormones does not correct it.

Abnormal blood flow certainly is important in cognitive functions. After a concussion people have a hard time focusing and remembering, even if there was no structural damage to the brain. As in migraine, abnormal function of the blood vessels may play a critical role.

Unfortunately this vasculopathy cannot be seen under the microscope. But while there is no pathology to see on a dead piece of tissue under the microscope, the blood vessels do not function normally, and in nearly every area searched, abnormalities are found. This is because the chemistry that rules blood vessel function is abnormal. And it is likely that nitric oxide and acetylcholine are central.

Traditionally we have wanted to say that the blood vessels are too dilated or large; or on the other hand, they are too constricted or small. In neuro-immune fatigue they are both, again adding to the confusion. But the role of dysregulated nitric oxide as a mediator in this area suggests a possible answer. Nitric oxide by itself is a vasodilator – it opens up blood vessels and makes them floppy. But the floppy, dilated vessels cause the adrenals to compensate with adrenalin to constrict the vessels. Furthermore, nitric oxide is converted to superoxide which is a vasoconstrictor. Overall, the excess production of nitric oxide or the inability to get rid of it safely leads to the equivalent of a blood vessel nervous breakdown, a vasculopathy. Let us review a few studies related to abnormalities within the vascular system.

## Blood Pressure

A persons' blood pressure is a general measure of the pressure to circulate blood throughout the body. Because elevated blood pressure is linked to heart disease and stroke, there has been a great deal of attention in trying to reduce it to make people healthier. While this is true of heart disease, it may be that for some persons with ME/CFS, the blood pressure is too low.

It is ironic that when a healthy-looking person walks into the doctor's office with a blood pressure of 75/40, medical providers think that everything is fine. But if a patient in the intensive care unit were to have the same blood pressure, sirens would go off all over the place. Blood pressure is the result of the force of the heartbeat, the amount of blood in the body, and the size of the blood vessels. In order to get blood to the brain while standing up, it is necessary to have adequate blood pressure.

In general, most persons with ME/CFS have low blood pressure, but not all. A few ME/CFS patients will have high blood pressure which characteristically fluctuates. I think it is likely that the hypertension may result from the excessive constriction of blood vessels in an attempt to improve blood flow to the body. The constriction of the blood vessels may be due to adrenalin and can be measured. Historically we have called those persons as having "hyperaderenergic orthostatic intolerance" where the levels of blood vessel constrictors are measured to be high. One interesting phenomenon is "orthostatic diastolic hypertension" where the bottom number of the blood pressure rises to an abnormal level when a person with ME/CFS stands up. Normally it should stay the same or even drop.

<u>Circulating Blood Volume</u>

Back in 1995 I had the good fortune of meeting Dr. David Streeten for the first time. He was a professor of medicine in Syracuse, New York, and had been studying "delayed orthostatic hypotension". It quickly became clear to us that we were both studying the same illness, and we joined forces. His work revolved around orthostatic intolerance, and the reduction in blood flow to the brain while standing. He would have a patient lie quietly on the examining table for twenty minutes with readings of pulse and blood pressure, then stand the patient by the bedside and continuously monitor pulse and blood pressure. He noted several abnormal patterns, but the one he was most interested in was "delayed orthostatic hypotension", meaning that the blood pressure would begin to drop after a while and the patient would come close to fainting. This response is quite different from that of the normal fainter.

He had made the observation that these patients had a reduction in circulating blood volume, and we went on to study twenty-five patients and published a paper with the results (Streeten-2000). The amount of blood circulating within the body stays relatively constant at 70 mL per kilogram of body weight. Thus for a 200 lb man, the amount of blood coursing through his vascular system should be more than 5 quarts. People who live at the top of a mountain will have a little more because they need to carry more oxygen. Dehydrated people in the desert will have a little less, but the body is very good at maintaining blood volume even under adverse conditions.

To measure the blood volume is simple, but is not done on standard tests; it must be performed in a nuclear medicine laboratory. A tube of blood is taken and the red blood cells and serum albumin are separated and tagged. The blood is then given back to the patient, allowed to circulate for a while and a new sample is drawn. The amount of tag on the red blood cells will be measured and indicate the total red blood cell mass; the albumin tag indicates the plasma volume. Added together they measure the circulating blood volume. Someone who is anemic will have a low red blood cell mass but normal or increased plasma volume, thus leading to a normal total blood volume. Someone dehydrated will have a normal red blood cell mass but a low plasma volume. Nearly 70% of patients with ME/ CFS, will have a reduction in circulating blood volume (Streeten-2000; Hurwitz-2007 IACFS conference).

This reduction in red cell mass implies a chronic situation, not an acute loss of blood. In some patients we have performed several measurements; they don't seem to change much. We looked at the mechanisms which the body uses to regulate circulating blood volume and they all seem to be working, although antidiuretic hormone is sluggish. So why is there a reduction in the circulating blood volume?

I think the answer lies in the vasculopathy. Think of the blood vessels as pipes in a building. If the pipes are small, the total volume of fluid in all the pipes of the building will be reduced. A normal blood volume assumes normal sized pipes, but if the blood vessels were constricted, then the total volume would be less. And indeed, some of our patients have a dramatic reduction in blood volume, some to about 50% of normal. That's 2 ½ quarts down all the time. In a car accident, if you lose half of your blood volume it is fatal, but in ME/CFSFM this reduction is not due to a sudden blood loss, as in bleeding. In its own sick way, the body seems to get used to it, sort of.

But nitric oxide is a vasodilator in itself. If the circulating blood volume of a person with neuro-immune fatigue is reduced, could this be a result of the body's attempt to establish vasoconstrictor tone? Or could it be the nitric oxide by-products that act as vasoconstrictors? As present, these areas have not been explored, but they could lead to more effective sub grouping in the research setting.

Orthostatic Intolerance

This term refers to the inability of a person to tolerate the upright position, primarily because the brain does not get enough blood when in the upright position. While orthostatic intolerance has been defined in different ways, I feel that nearly everyone with neuro-immune fatigue has some degree of it. This is the reason persons will be overcome with exhaustion while walking out to get the mail. Or a person will feel lightheaded and almost faint while standing at the checkout counter of the supermarket. Or a person needs a chair while taking a hot shower. One person said that he had "paralyzing fatigue", yet because he looked healthy to the medical provider they assumed he was a fruitcake. What cannot be seen by the medical provider is the amount of blood in the brain at a given time.

There have been numerous studies now demonstrating orthostatic intolerance in neuro-immune fatigue. Combined with the measured reduction in circulating blood volume, the question remains as to whether the symptoms of ME/CFS/FM are due to decreased cerebral blood flow in the upright position.

One of the first attempts to answer this was to increase circulating blood volume with fludrocortisone, an adrenal steroid which acts by holding onto salt and water in the kidneys. While the early studies by Drs. Rowe and colleagues at Johns Hopkins were encouraging (Rowe-95), it has not worked out as well as initially hoped. Adding a medication (midodrine) to constrict the blood vessels of the lower extremities and thus increase cerebral blood flow may help a bit, but not much. Also, the midodrine is poorly tolerated, presumably because the adrenergic system is already maxed out.

Dr. David Streeten did a fascinating study on some of my patients. He stood them up, and, as with nearly all patients with ME/CFS/FM, they tolerate quiet standing poorly. He then compressed the body with something called MAST trousers (for Military Anti-Shock Trousers) which force the blood to the central organs of heart, lungs, and brain. Patients with this external pressure could stand without the symptoms of the orthostatic intolerance (Streeten-00).

The trousers are very bulky and you cannot move with then on. However one of my patients purchased a set and would get propped up at the sink so she could do the dishes. Yes, it shows that the orthostatic intolerance is improved with MAST trousers, but more importantly, it shows how desperate patients with neuro-immune fatigue can be to return to the routine activities of daily life. Another type of orthostatic intolerance is POTS (postural orthostatic tachycardia syndrome) and

Julian Stewart's work indicates it may be due to reduced blood flow through the heart and lungs (Stewart-04).

Cerebral Blood Flow

The critical issue here is the amount of blood in the brain. There are technical difficulties in measuring the amount of blood that happens to be in the brain at any given moment. Archimedes could have solved this problem by removing the patient's head and seeing how much water it displaces, but this technique will not get past current ethics committees. Primary care physicians would be eager to have such a study done as it would solve their "problem" with patients who take up so much of their time. There have been many brain blood flow studies that have showed abnormal distribution of blood flow in neuro-immune fatigue.

One recent study has measured absolute brain blood flow and shown it to be both lower than normal and different from patients who had primary depression (Yoshiuchi-06). In another study an attempt was made to correlate the reduced cerebral blood flow to the severity of fatigue. The blood flow pattern was abnormal, but no association was found between fatigue levels and cerebral perfusion. This makes the routine use of SPECT scans less valuable (Fischler-96). Furthermore, it implies that while a vasculopathy may be present, it is not the sole explanation for the severity of fatigue, an important factor that we will look at later.

So far there have been no studies adequately explaining the poor cerebral blood flow, but one interesting finding has been noted in patients with orthostatic intolerance. In this study Julian Stewart measured levels of angiotensin II, known to constrict the blood vessels of the brain and other vessels of the body and found it to be high. He also correlated this to low brain blood flow and a reduction in the body's circulating blood volume (Stewart-06). This suggests that because of a reduction in the circulating blood volume in the body, the body tries to compensate by producing adrenalin and other blood vessel constrictors to improve the flow. Unfortunately it does not really help as it can further reduce blood flow by narrowing the pipes. This may be why a large group of neuro-immune fatigue patients (usually the most severe) do not do well with coffee and stimulants which further constrict the blood vessels. It is possible that this is represents an important subgroup and that those without the secondary vasoconstriction can be treated effectively with vasoconstrictors.

<u>Cognitive impairment</u>

Reduced blood flow to the brain will certainly cause cognitive difficulties. Ask any intensive care nurse; when a person's blood pressure is falling they cannot think clearly. The cognitive abnormalities in this illness are complex, and unlikely to be due entirely to reduced blood flow. However a few observations suggest that the flow is an important issue.

If you ask healthy people how they read their magazines or books they usually state that they read at a table or sitting in an armchair. Persons with ME/CFS/FM usually read lying down. It is likely that with the legs elevated, blood flow to the brain is improved and they will have improved concentration. Studies of cognitive function have not taken orthostatic intolerance into account, and it would be interesting to do a study of cognitive skills after resting and after standing for fifteen minutes.

The question is not trivial. One of the many unanswered questions is whether the cognitive abnormalities of persons with ME/CFS/FM are permanent or reversible. If the cognitive impairments are related to orthostatic intolerance either in whole or in part, several treatment regimens are suggested. Again, this remains to be tested.

<u>Blood Flow to Muscles</u>

In a preliminary study which is of interest because it relates to both vascular flow and cellular hypoxia, six ME/CFS patients and eight healthy persons exercised to exhaustion while a specific muscle was examined for blood flow and metabolic changes. Oxygen saturation was altered in the muscle of ME/CFS patients, implying abnormalities in energy metabolism as well as a reduction in total blood flow to the muscle (Neary-06). These results imply a simultaneous problem with both blood flow and energy production. Blood flow to muscles is a central topic in fibromyalgia research, and numerous treatments such as massage and heat attempt to relieve the muscle discomfort by increasing blood flow.

Blood flow in the legs is abnormal in persons with neuro-immune fatigue. Observations have been made of a blue discoloration of the feet implying pooling of the venous blood in the dependent position. Dr. Streeten infused vasoconstrictors into the veins of the feet and noted that the responses of the blood vessels were abnormal with impaired venous tone (Streeten-96).

In an important study to help define the vasculopathy, Dr. Vance Spence measured the blood vessels for their responses to acetylcholine, a vasodilator closely related to nitric oxide. He noted that the vasodilation remains longer in ME/CFS than in controls. Importantly, his group noted differences between those with "classic" ME/CFS/FM and those with Gulf war illness, presumable related to exposure to pesticides (Khan-04). This demonstrated that the overall picture of the symptoms may be similar even with different cellular mechanisms in place. The details of the vasculopathy have yet to be demonstrated in detail, particularly in different subgroups of patients, but the existence of a widespread problem in blood vessel function has been established.

Conclusion

There is ample evidence now that blood flow to heart, muscles and brain is abnormal in ME/CFS/FM. However, correcting regional blood flow does little to improve the overall symptom pattern in my experience. The vasculopathy is a process that exists and can be demonstrated, but is not the major disabling feature of ME/CFS. The vasculopathy has been a confusing side issue; present but of uncertain significance. Too bad because it is one group of symptoms that may be most promising to treat.

Nitric oxide dysregulation is a very logical candidate to account for the vasculopathy. However, because of the daunting problems in research in this area, studies showing the "smoking gun" are lacking. But I have great hope that attention is turning to this area now.

References

Fischler B, D'Haenen H, Cluydts R, Michiels V, Demets K, Bossuyt A, et al. Comparison of 99m Tc HMPAO SPECT scan between chronic fatigue syndrome, major depression and healthy controls: an exploratory study of clinical correlates of regional cerebral blood flow. Neuropsychobiology 1996;34:175-183

Gerrity T, Bates J, Bell D, Chrousos G, Furst G, Hedrick T, Hurwitz B, Kula RW, Levine SM, Moore RC, Schondorf R. Chronic fatigue syndrome: What role does the autonomic nervous system play in the pathophysiology of this complex illness? Neuroimmunomodulation 2002;10:134-141.

Khan F, Kennedy G, Spence V, Newton D, Belch J: Peripheral cholinergic function in humans with chronic fatigue syndrome, Gulf War syndrome and with illness following organophosphate exposure. *Clin Sci* 2004, 106:183-189

Murad F. Nitric oxide and cyclic GMP in cell signaling and drug development. N Eng J Med 2006;355:2003-2011

Neary J, Roberts A, Leavins N, Harrison M, Croll J, Sexsmith J, et al. Muscle hemodynamics and oxygen saturation during exercise in chronic fatigue syndrome patients. Medicine & Science in Sports and Exercise 2006;38(5):S359.

Rowe P, Bou-Holaigh I, Kan J, Calkins H: Is neurally mediated hypotension an unrecognized cause of chronic fatigue? *Lancet* 1995, 345:623-625

Stewart J, Glover J, MS M. Increased plasma angiotensin II in postural tachycardia syndrome (POTS) is related to reduced blood flow and blood volume. Clin Sci 2006;110(2):255-263

Stewart J, Montgomery L. Regional blood volume and peripheral blood flow in postural tachycardia syndrome. Am HJ Physiol Heart Circ Physiol 2004;287:H1319-H1327.

Streeten D, Thomas D, Bell D. The roles of orthostatic hypotension, orthostatic tachycardia, and subnormal erythrocyte volume in the pathogenesis of the chronic fatigue syndrome. American Journal of the Medical Sciences 2000;320(1):1-8.

Streeten DHP, Scullard TF. Excessive gravitational blood pooling caused by impaired venous tone is the predominant non-cardiac mechanism of orthostatic intolerance. Clin Sci (Colch) 1996; 90: 277-285.

Yoshiuchi K, Farkas J, Natelson B. Patients with chronic fatigue syndrome have reduced absolute blood flow. Clin Physiol Funct Imaging 2006;26:83-86.

# Chapter 9: Symptom Cluster #2: Central Sensitization

The neuro-immune spectrum of illnesses is nowhere as diverse as in the subject of central sensitization, yet it plays an important role in each condition. Central sensitization means a central nervous system that is "sensitized"; it is a disorder of the ability of the central nervous system to modulate sensory input.

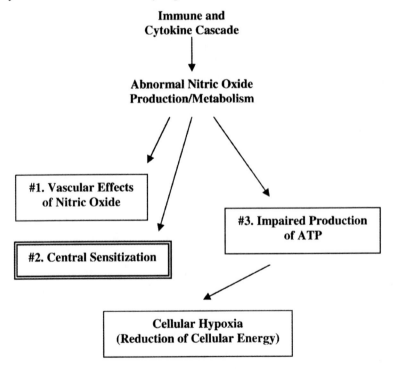

**Immune and Cytokine Cascade**

**Abnormal Nitric Oxide Production/Metabolism**

**#1. Vascular Effects of Nitric Oxide**

**#2. Central Sensitization**

**#3. Impaired Production of ATP**

**Cellular Hypoxia (Reduction of Cellular Energy)**

My father would have said that the nervous system "is on the Fritz". I never knew what a Fritz actually was, but in the illnesses we are talking about the nerves are there.

The first and probably most prominent symptom is pain. In ME/CFS/FM (and all the illnesses under this umbrella) there is an abnormal perception of sensory stimuli, likely from two separate but related mechanisms. The first mechanism is increased amplitude of the nerve impulses, and the second is a decreased ability to dampen or modulate them.

The pain of ME/CFS/FM is everywhere: headache, eyes ache, muscle and joint pain, sore throat, lymph node pain. Sometimes the pain is so severe and widespread that the skin and hair hurt – called allodynia. The section of the neuro-immune spectrum called fibromyalgia is particularly famous for pain, a dubious distinction at best.

And if you take a biopsy of anyplace where pain is perceived and study it under a microscope, there is no tissue damage to be found. Of course people have jumped to the conclusion that patients with these conditions were fruitcakes and were making up the pain. Hypochondriacs, wimps and fruitcakes (don't get me started). We now know this is not true. The pain is not from classical tissue damage, but from the inability of the nervous system to transmit and modulate the nerve impulses accurately.

A second area of central sensitization is in the increased perceived intensity of light and noise. Persons with ME/CFS/FM sometimes wear sunglasses inside the house. Night driving is difficult because of glare. The noise of the television in the background is unpleasant. For a few, the noise sensitivity is the most disabling symptom, requiring earmuffs and a sound-proof room, and I have two or three patients where this occurs.

All sensory input into the nervous system can be unpleasant. This is one of the minor symptoms of the illness that indicates both illness severity and the likelihood of resolution. Central sensitization is the reason that patients with ME/CFS/FM will describe the mall as hell on earth. In the mall, particularly at Christmas time, there is lots of noise, bright lights, and commotion – people running around. Add to this mix a little orthostatic intolerance and you have a description of hell. Merry Christmas.

Another area of central sensitization is increased sensitivity to temperature changes. Hot flashes and chills at strange times, sweats that make no sense. Most persons with neuro-immune fatigue are heat intolerant, some cold intolerant and medical providers look toward the thyroid for an explanation. A poorly recognized part of this symptom cluster is a generalized anxiety, and sensory myoclonus. The anxiety is routinely said to be psychological, but it may actually be a neurologic symptom lodged within this cluster. A number of my patients have a form of myoclonic seizures which are extreme examples.

It is not uncommon for excessive reflexes. Normally, when the knee is hit by the reflex hammer, the input goes to the spine and down to the muscles of the leg, causing it to jerk. In persons with the more severe form of ME/CFS/FM, the impulse spreads and the whole body jerks. This is called sensory stimulus myoclonus, and is an example of the nervous system being unable to modulate the impulses correctly.

Central sensitization is another daunting subject, only recently beginning to expose itself to medical understanding. Studies to measure it and seek its biochemistry are only now beginning to expand.

Pain

The central nervous system normally is confronted with a dilemma. It has to notify, experience, and record sensory input so that the brain can learn from the environment in which it lives. We step on a thorn; we learn from the experience. By learning, it helps us prevent or limit the damage. In a very real way we need pain. My gym teacher would love to hear me say that now.

However, if we do step on a thorn, at a certain point the brain needs to say "OK, I know about this pain, now let's forget it and move on." The pain should not be continuous, but should lessen and eventually stop; otherwise it no longer serves a purpose. A finger is caught in a mousetrap. It hurts like crazy for a while then gets less and less. This is called modulation. The central nervous system modifies the sensory input and it decreases.

Patients with neuro-immune fatigue are remarkable in how poorly this system works. I learned this in 1990 with a mitochondria/muscle biopsy study done by Dr. June Aprille. I informed my ten patients that muscle biopsies hurt, and they all agreed to the research and signed informed consent. The biopsies were small clean cuts into the muscle, numbed with Novocain. They all healed well without infection. But the pain from this procedure exceeded anything I expected to hear. One patient said she had lingering pain at the site six months later.

The abnormal perception of pain is important for medical providers to understand in neuro-immune fatigue. If you assess a condition by the amount of pain, as in a slipped disc of the back, you may be more likely to have surgery. And instead of reducing the pain it will only intensify it.

In ME/CFS/FM there are two problems with this system broadly under the term central sensitization. The first problem is that the threshold for pain is lowered. Something that should not hurt is now perceived as painful. In its most extreme form (in ME/CFS/FM as well as migraine and other illnesses with central sensitization) is allodynia. Touching the skin is perceived as painful. The second problem is that the responsiveness to the stimulus is increased. Added together, sensory stimuli can be very uncomfortable. The nervous system is normally a marvelous design and can adapt and change: it has plasticity. Sometimes that plasticity can go haywire.

Wind-up pain

There are two arms within central sensitization that we will examine. The first is wind-up pain, or central afferent pain amplification. Studied now for a number of years, it has been noticed that if a repeated stimulus is applied, there is a gradual increase in the perception of pain. It is as if the pain is "winding up." The type of nerve fibers which transmit regular and wind up pain are different, which is the reason certain medications will not help with this latter type of pain. It is this wind-up pain that is prominent in ME/CFS/FM.

The mechanism of wind up pain is felt to be due to activation of NMDA receptors. This receptor activation induces calcium to enter into cells and activates the nitric oxide synthetase system. This, in turn, causes the release of peptides that increase pain sensation, including substance P. Substance P acts by lowering the threshold of membrane excitability, and the wind-up becomes a vicious cycle (Meeus and Nijs-07).

It has long been known that a specific injury or repeated injury can lead to generalized pain. This is the bad news; what starts as localized or regional pain such as whiplash of a slipped disc in the back can evolve into widespread pain. Persistent localized moderate to severe pain can induce generalization of severe pain and its permanence. It can become generalized fibromyalgia (Henriksson 03).

## Reduced Pain Modulation

The second arm of central sensitization is impaired pain inhibition. Think of a nerve as a piano wire. It is struck by the hammer and vibrates to create a sound. But the pianist may want the sound to be dampened and so steps on the middle pedal of the piano. This presses against the wire to reduce the vibration and thus decreases the sound. The body has its middle pedal and it is called inhibitory control.

Normally this system is effective and necessary to remove nervous system "noise". In neuro-immune fatigue the inhibitory control does not function well and the noise becomes painful. All noise, meaning sensory stimuli – odors, commotion, light, touch, and sound. It is possible to diagnose persons in the movie theater who have neuro-immune fatigue because they have sunglasses on and cotton sticking out of their ears.

There is an overlap between what we are calling the symptom cluster of central sensitization and the vasculopathy symptom cluster. There is reduced blood perfusion in many tissues. This reduced blood flow may cause a reduced tissue oxygen level which will itself cause the activation of the nitric oxide system. It has also been suggested that the altered hypothalamic-pituitary-adrenal (HPA) axis may be important, as estrogen levels also influence pain. There have been numerous recent reviews of pain mechanisms (McCabe-04), but so far researchers have been unsuccessful in differentiating the illnesses of the neuro-immune fatigue spectrum, probably because these mechanisms are cellular and not organ specific.

## Peripheral sensory abnormalities

As in the discussion of immunity, it is becoming clear that there are peripheral abnormalities also involved in the abnormal pain perception. In one interesting study, Leonardo Vecchiet and co-workers showed selective muscle hypersensitivity related to enzyme abnormalities in muscle mitochondria. This would imply that there is both central and peripheral pain processing difficulties present in

*David S. Bell MD, FAAP*

ME/CFS (Vecchiet-96). However, we should not be surprised that both central and peripheral tissues are involved because the problem exists in every cell of the body.

Conclusions

The presence of an abnormality within the central nervous system is beginning to stand alone as an explanation for the widespread pain and sensitivities of ME/CFS/FM. Moreover, a central role for nitric oxide in this explanation is evolving as well. If nitric oxide is responsible for one group of symptoms because it dilates blood vessels, why shouldn't it cause another group of symptoms in its actions as a neurotransmitter? One of the problems with a cellular chemical as basic as nitric oxide is that when it is not right (on the Fritz) it will show up in different areas. In fact, if one looks at the many diverse functions of nitric oxide one sees the clinical picture of the conditions within the neuro-immune spectrum.

References

Bengtsson M, Bengtsson A, Jorfeldt L. Diagnostic epidural opioid blockade in primary fibromyalgia at rest and during exercise. Pain. 1989; 39:171-180

McCabe C. Pain mechanisms and the rheumatic diseases. Musculoskeletal Care 2004;2(2):75-89

Henriksson K. Hypersensitivity in muscle pain syndromes. Current Pain and Headache Reports 2003;7:426-432

Meeus M, Nijs J. Central sensitization: a bio-psychosocial explanation for chronic widespread pain in patients with fibromyalgia and chronic fatigue syndrome. *Clin Rheumatol* 2007, 26(4):465-473.

Mountz JM, Bradley LA, Modell JG et al. Fibromyalgia in women: abnormalities of regional cerebral blood flow in the thalamus and the caudate nucleus are associated with low pain threshold levels. Arthritis Rheum. 1995; 38:926-938

Vecchiet L, Montanari G, Pizzigallo E, et al: Sensory characterization of somatic parietal tissues in humans with chronic fatigue syndrome. *Neurosci Lett* 1996, 208:117-120.

# Chapter 10: Symptom Cluster #3: Cytopathic Hypoxia

At this point it appears that some of the bricks are falling into place. We have a cellular explanation of some of the symptoms in the vascular and central nervous systems, but we still do not have an adequate explanation for fatigue. And the activity limitation due to fatigue and exhaustion is probably the most critical symptom in this whole spectrum of illnesses.

We can temporarily correct the orthostatic hypotension. The patient can lie in a comfortable position for several days so the blood flow to the brain is well established, but the symptoms do not entirely go away. We can abolish postural tachycardia with different therapeutic techniques and medications but the symptom pattern remains. It may be slightly improved, but it is still there. We can correct the reduced circulating blood volume with erythropoietin, plasma infusions, saline and blood transfusion, but again, the symptom pattern is still present. The central sensitization is much harder to correct, but pain medications and anti-seizure medications (which raise the impulse threshold) may have a little benefit. As a patient of mine once said, "It is possible to treat the symptoms, but the illness remains." By this she meant the exhaustion, malaise, and fatigue.

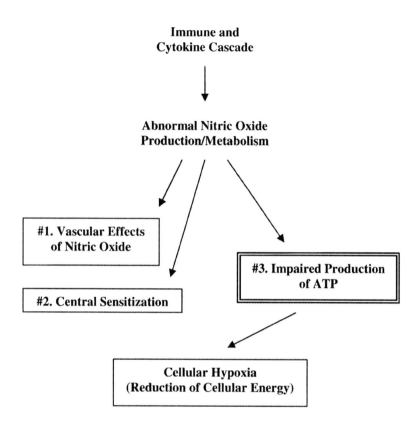

If the vasculopathy and central sensitization are related to nitric oxide effects, what else does nitric oxide do that could give us a hint? The cardiovascular effects of nitric oxide include vasodilator tone, stimulating growth of blood vessels, and inhibiting platelet activation. In the nervous system it regulates sensory perception, acts in the brain as a neurotransmitter affecting memory and other functions, and it affects peripheral nerve transmission in the intestine and bladder. In the immune system it affects natural killer cells, cytotoxicity, and programmed cell death. All of these details seem to be present in the neuro-immune fatigue spectrum, but they are all just confusing details, almost of no importance to the primary disabling symptom. We call this symptom fatigue for lack of a better term. Exhaustion, malaise, dysphoria, asthenia, weakness all apply. My patients would say they feel like crap.

It turns out that nitric oxide has another important effect in the area of metabolism. It impairs energy production by the cell. Without adequate energy production, everything in the body starts to slow down. If you have a piece of muscle without energy, it is said to experience muscle fatigue. You need energy in the form of ATP (adenosine triphosphate) to make proteins, to think, to digest food properly, and to transmit messages along nerves. ATP is the energy produced by cellular metabolism that runs the body. It is our gasoline, and without it, everything stops.

It turns out that nitric oxide impairs the production of ATP in several ways. It can directly block access of oxygen to the machinery of the energy production system. It can stimulate poly ADP ribose polymerase-1 which affects NADPH to reduce energy utilization. But, perhaps more importantly, when nitric oxide is degraded it turns into two very nasty toxic by-products, superoxide and peroxynitrite. These two chemicals under normal conditions are removed safely from the body by being transformed into hydrogen peroxide and water. But under abnormal conditions they poison the mitochondria, the energy manufacturing machinery of the cell.

And this is the bottom line. Without energy the body experiences fatigue. Without energy the body cannot carry out normal maintenance. And with poisoned mitochondria the body feels sick. Overall we call this process cellular hypoxia, the inability of the cell to turn oxygen and glucose into energy and carbon dioxide. So now our diagram looks like this:

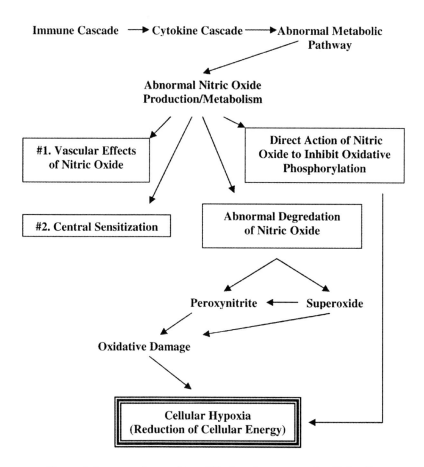

One of the great joys of my life has been to make little diagrams like this.

### Mitochondria

As we discussed earlier, mitochondria are small energy producing packets within the cell. There are between three and five hundred mitochondria in any given cell, more in brain and muscle cells where lots of energy is needed, and less in tissues like bone. Mitochondria take in oxygen and glucose and transform these building blocks into energy (ATP) and carbon dioxide. Mitochondrial abnormalities in ME/CFS/FM have been hypothesized for many years, but it is only recently that they are being demonstrated. Earlier concepts of mitochondrial disease required complete failure of mitochondria with abnormal mitochondrial DNA, but with ME/CFS/FM the sub-cellular structure is normal; it is in the biochemistry that the production of energy impaired. Genetic mitochondrial disease is often fatal in childhood whereas ME/CFS/FM is acquired, can resolve on its own, and has normal mitochondrial DNA.

One interesting example of abnormal mitochondrial function is due to lack of thyroid hormone, or hypothyroidism. The similarities between ME/CFS/FM and hypothyroidism are well known and some clinicians try to treat the illness with high doses of thyroid hormone. The reason the illnesses are so similar is that when thyroid hormone is reduced, the oxidative phosphorylation, the production of ATP, is reduced. This occurs at a slightly different place within the mitochondria from what is going on with ME/CFS/FM, but the reduction of temperature, energy, and other symptoms is similar.

And here is the paradigm shift that is necessary to understand ME/ CFS/FM. We say that thyroid disease is due to a poorly functioning organ, the thyroid. We could as well say that thyroid disease is a mitochondrial disease. In neuro-immune fatigue we have no localizing organ such as the thyroid on which to place the blame, and as a result of the confusion, some people say that the illness doesn't exist or isn't real. But it is as real as hypothyroidism.

The mechanism within the mitochondria that does the actual transformation of chemical energy is called oxidative phosphorylation. It is a complex process (another damn cascade) that takes the energy from food and transfers it down a line of enzymatic reactions until it is stored as a high energy phosphate bond. ADP becomes ATP. The ATP can then be taken to where ever it is needed. When energy is needed for a specific function, the high energy bond is broken and ATP again becomes ADP. I visualize it as a bunch of little suitcases carrying tiny amounts of plutonium. Because the chain is long and complex, there are many places where it can fail or be blocked. As we described the mitochondria earlier as round dinner tables scattered throughout the ballroom, we would now have to say that the ATP would be little radioactive, mouse-sized lunchboxes coming out of the table.

And where does mitochondrial dysfunction fit in into the neuro-immune fatigue spectrum? In a recent genomics paper by Susan

Vernon and co-workers the issue is addressed directly: "We found that individuals who suffered from post-infective fatigue had a distinct gene expression profile during the acute illness compared to those whose illness resolved. Evaluation of the gene expression profile over the course of the year implicated an altered host response to EBV and mitochondrial dysfunction in those who developed post-infective fatigue." They go on to state, "Our preliminary results implicate mitochondrial dysfunction as a plausible physiologic perturbation in post-infective fatigue." (Vernon-06)

In very general terms, this mitochondrial dysfunction is cellular hypoxia. Cellular hypoxia is a term meaning oxygen starvation within the cell. Most commonly hypoxia refers to the cell not getting oxygen from the blood stream, but in this case the blood has plenty of oxygen and it gets to the cell (although sometimes poorly). The problem is that the mitochondria cannot turn it into energy properly. And with the energy chain "uncoupled" oxygen can get to the cell, it may even get to the mitochondria, but adequate energy is not produced. Oxidative phosphorylation is like a long freight train, and huge segments of the train get uncoupled and lie stranded on the tracks. Even I am getting confused by these metaphors.

Oxidative stress is a term used to describe changes caused by prolonged exposure to a greater concentration of free radicals (oxyradicals) than can be neutralized by the body. Free radicals are part of the normal by-products of cellular metabolism, chemicals such as peroxynitrite and superoxide. These free radicals, also known as oxidants, can be neutralized by "antioxidants" such as some enzyme systems, vitamins and other cellular substrates. Antioxidants are part of the normal defense mechanism of the cell. Reactive oxygen species (ROS), another term for oxyradicals, and other oxidants can also affect lipid membranes causing changes in membrane function. Mitochondria may be particularly sensitive to oxidative damage both by damage to the mitochondrial membrane and to the respiratory chain. Damage to mitochondrial components, including the membranes, impairs their ability to produce ATP. One of the possible reasons for the variations within the spectrum of neuro-immune fatigue is that there are so many places within the cellular structures where cellular hypoxia may occur.

Furthermore, all the conditions in this spectrum are chronic by definition. There is no simple damage and then healing. Because of the fundamental nature of nitric oxide metabolism in the cells, particularly in the immune system, once this abnormal cascade begins, it does not want to turn itself off. The title of one recent paper summarizes the phenomenon: "Antiviral pathway deregulation of chronic fatigue syndrome induces nitric oxide production that precludes a resolution of the inflammatory response" (Fremont-06)

## Proof

Ah..... Here comes both the bad news and the greatest hope for the future. First the bad news. What is being described here sounds easy to prove but is not. No one has ever looked at the whole neuro-immune spectrum with a consistent plan to measure cellular hypoxia. The emphasis has been to break down and sub-classify illnesses such as chronic fatigue syndrome with meticulous diagnostic criteria and study that small portion. But the methods used with one portion are going to be different from that used in the other portions. Even within a small and well-defined portion there may be twenty subcategories and the labyrinth just goes deeper. Furthermore, as discussed in the introduction, our focus has been on organs not cellular structures. I am not sure we even know how to study energy production by the body as a whole.

In one interesting study patients with ME/CFS had muscle biopsies looking for enterovirus, one of the candidate viruses known to initiate the illness in some patients. Of the 48 patients in the study, 21% were positive for enterovirus, again reflecting the topic we discussed earlier. All the patients had exercise testing prior to the biopsy. Of the ten patients who were positive for enterovirus infection, nine had an abnormal lactate production with exercise, demonstrating abnormal energy production. This would directly imply an abnormality of mitochondria in the muscles (Lane-2003).

The medical literature is enormously complex on the subject of energy production and oxidative damage in different disease states. There are now at least fifty papers within the neuro-immune fatigue area, most of them clearly demonstrating the presence of both reduced energy production and oxidative damage.

But there has been one remarkable set of studies which may have found a smoking gun. Drs. Mark Van Ness, Chris Snell and Staci Stevens of the

University of the Pacific focused on the post-exertional malaise, perhaps the central distinguishing symptom of ME/CFS, in an attempt to demonstrate the effects of exertion on exercise tolerance. Six patients exercised while being measured for oxygen consumption and carbon dioxide release on two consecutive days. The first day test showed reduced exercise ability, a finding noted on many tests of this type, and often inappropriately attributed to deconditioning. But when tested the following day with the same exercise, the patients did much worse, demonstrating the post-exertional malaise. The worsening was due to a change in anaerobic threshold, a reduced ability of the cells to utilize oxygen in aerobic metabolism. The exercise of the first day caused a poisoning of the mitochondria which showed up on the exercise test of day two.

The reason that day one exercise is poor is that persons with neuro-immune fatigue normally restrict their activity to conserve energy, and not because they are lazy. The low values of anaerobic threshold are an attempt to compensate for the illness, and are not due to deconditioning. In lazy persons or fruitcakes (they are different) there is no change in the anaerobic threshold on the second day of exercise.

In this study control, sedentary patients improved their anaerobic threshold from 17.5 to 18. In ME/CFS patients they started somewhat lower, at 15, and dropped to 11. The only explanation for this decrease is a change in the ability of the cells to utilize oxygen and produce energy (Van Ness-06).

This study emphasizes a fact that all patients with ME/CFS/FM know from experience. If you test a cellular system in this illness under resting conditions, the results are not so far off. If you ask a person with emphysema to read an article, it is not too abnormal. But if you stress the system with exercise you will bring out the abnormalities. Ask the person with emphysema to run around the block.

Thus to demonstrate the energy production abnormalities, in the future it will be critical to test mitochondrial metabolism and function when the system is stressed. A muscle biopsy for mitochondria taken after a patient has been resting for three days is likely to be quite different from a biopsy taken after exercise. The stress does not have to be limited to exercise, but can be neuronal or immune activation or medications known to affect the metabolic pathways. The area of potential research in this area is virtually endless, and will lead to the mechanisms that can then be treated.

## Conclusions

We have seen how it is possible that nitric oxide deregulation can affect the vascular and central nervous systems. But another known problem with nitric oxide is that it can block the production of cellular energy in several different ways. Some blocks are due to a direct action of nitric oxide on the ATP production machinery, and some are from the toxic metabolites of nitric oxide breakdown.

So far the research on the abnormal energy metabolism of neuro-immune fatigue has been piecemeal. What is needed is the same approach that occurs when a patient goes to the medical provider with a cut that does not stop bleeding. The provider measures the twenty or more different steps in the blood-clotting cascade to find the problem. Then an appropriate treatment can be applied.

## References

Fink M. Bench-to-bedside review: Cytopathic hypoxia. Critical Care 2002;6:491-499.

Fremont M, Vaeyens F, Herst CV, De Meirleir K, Englebienne P. Antiviral pathway deregulation of chronic fatigue syndrome induces nitric oxide production that precludes a resolution of the inflammatory response. JCFS; 13(4):17-28.

Lane R, Soteriou B, Zhang H, Archard L. Enterovirus related metabolic myopathy: a postviral fatigue syndrome. J Neurol Neurosurg Psychiatry 2003;74:1382-1386

VanNess J, Snell C, Stevens S, Bateman L, Keller B. Using serial cardiopulmonary exercise tests to support a diagnosis of chronic fatigue syndrome. Medicine & Science in Sports and Exercise 2006;38(5):S85

Vernon S, Whistler T, Cameron B, Hickie I, Reeves W, Lloyd A. Preliminary evidence of mitochondrial dysfunction associated with post-infectious fatigue after acute infection with Epstein-Barr virus. BMC Infectious Diseases 2006;6: http://www.biomedcentral.com/1471-2334/1476/1416

# Chapter 11: Treatment Considerations

Well, we have covered some ground. If this monograph turns out to be even close to predicting the direction of the neuro-immune fatigue science of the future, good treatment should be just around the corner. And the hope for the future is profound. If we, as an educated and enlightened collection of nations can focus our resources upon health care, we will be able to accomplish this research.

It has been done before. In pediatrics there is a subspecialty of metabolic medicine. Each of the conditions studied in this subspecialty may be caused by a different enzyme abnormality, and each enzyme abnormality has its own clinical presentation and treatment. But at least there is a structure in place to start the work. And it has been effective in early diagnosis and treatment of conditions such as phenylketonuria (PKU).

The first step is accurate diagnosis. As with all illnesses, a good clinical history, physical examination and basic laboratory evaluation by compassionate and educated medical providers is the start. The second step would be an evaluation of nitric oxide production, and the ability of the body's enzyme systems to eliminate it, along with peroxynitrite and superoxide. The third step would be to evaluate the immune and metabolic cascades to discover the exact abnormality of an individual's symptoms.

Then comes treatment. We know of substances able to reduce the amount of nitric oxide within a system. Some of these substances, such as vitamin B12 have long been known and are safe. Some supplements, vitamins and drugs will be able to inhibit nitric oxide synthetase or improve the function of the enzyme systems to eliminate the reactive oxygen species. As has been done with the problem of too much cholesterol, research will discover the safest and most effective ways to correct the problem identified.

Already there are excellent clinicians offering treatments in these complex areas. Drs. Paul Cheney, Jacob Teitelbaum and Kenny DeMeirlier have been attempting to treat the metabolic abnormalities of neuro-immune fatigue for years. But the structure is not in place for their work to be standardized or reproduced

Accurate laboratory testing for 2'-5'A Synthetase, RNaseL, glutathione, catalase, nitric oxide, and the degree of oxidative stress is either not available, is not known to the average physician, or is not covered by medical insurance. And these are just the starters.

But I am optimistic. When I was in medical school we did not have the individual pieces of the blood clotting cascade. We never even heard of delta granule deficiency. And now we have not only the accurate steps of the cascade measured, it is covered by medical insurance, and treatments are available.

People say that it is too expensive to do testing and research in the metabolic areas of neuro-immune fatigue. But with the illnesses of this spectrum now being recognized more clearly, we can see that the social, medical, and economic costs are already staggering.

Years ago we embarked on a war on cancer. Neuro-immune fatigue can and will be conquered when we start to take it seriously. God willing, it can be done.